THE FIVE TRUTHS OF
TRANSFORMATIONAL WELLNESS
AND HOLISTIC HEALING

# TIMELESS YOU<sup>TH</sup>

Travis

Be well +

Live well!

DR. JEFF CRIPPEN, DC

innate press

This publication is designed to provide competent and reliable information regarding the subject matter covered. However, it is sold with the understanding that the author and publisher are not engaged in rendering medical, legal, financial, or other professional advice. Laws and practices often vary from state to state and country to country and if legal or other expert assistance is required, the services of a professional should be sought.

The stories in this book are based on actual patients. Certain identifying characteristics of patients, such as name, have been changed to respect their privacy.

Despite these changes, the arc of each patient's journey and the lessons learned by both patient and doctor are told faithfully. The author and publisher specifically disclaim any liability that is incurred from the use or application of the contents of this book. The publisher is not responsible for websites or their content that are not owned by the publisher.

Published by Innate Press, an imprint of Brisance Books Group, LLC.

Printed in Canada.

Hardcover Edition: November 2022
ISBN: 978-1-944194-85-7

Visit our website: CrippenWellness.com

112022

# DEDICATION

This book is dedicated to you...
those who are drawn to read it.

# HEALTH

1. The overall condition of an organism at a given time.

2. Soundness, especially of body or mind; freedom from disease or abnormality.

3. A condition of optimal well-being.

   From Indo-European root – meaning whole, uninjured, of good omen.

---

# PREFACE

Spanish explorer Juan Ponce de León was an adventurer at heart. He arrived in Florida in 1513 seeking fame and fortune through exploration. His days of exploration are believed to have begun in 1493, as part of Christopher Columbus's second expedition to the New World. However, on this trip to Florida, Ponce de León did not seek gold or silver. Instead, we are told, he was searching for the Fountain of Youth. The Fountain of Youth, the object of Ponce de León's search, was a miraculous spring that could rejuvenate anyone who drank from it. While its exact location has befuddled searchers, tales of its powers have been around for over 2,500 years. In fact, references to the healing waters of the Fountain of Youth go back to ancient Greece.

Ponce de León never found the Fountain of Youth. In fact, he died as a result of a subsequent trip to Florida. However, while he never found eternal youth, he did find fame as his name is still associated with the search for the Fountain of Youth.

Too often, when looking to create health, we look outside of ourselves. We look to the wisdom of doctors, or the magic of miracle drugs and trendy new supplements to help us tap into our own fountain of youth. But the truth is, the search for health will never be found by looking outside ourselves.

I know because I spent years searching.

What follows in the pages of *Timeless Youth* is a very personal account of my own journey. I was not looking for a fountain of youth, but searching instead to understand the true meaning of health so that I could live, and not suffer, through my own youth. I first fell ill when I was six years old, and then battled debilitating migraines for over a decade. These headaches with their chronic and overwhelming pain robbed me of many parts of my youth.

As my parents and I put our trust in well-credentialed doctors, FDA-approved prescription drugs, and the benefits of medical innovations to create health, ultimately I, like Ponce de León, never found what I was looking for.

Yet all along, the answer to my search was always within.

In fact, the word youth cannot be written without the letters y-o-u.

And it is within *you* that the secret to timeless youth is found.

Youth and you share the same root, *yeu* — which means vital force and youthful vigor. To create youth, we must, of course, radiate health.

This book, in a sense, is my own journey searching for the fountain of youth. However, rather than seeking a magical elixir found in the waters of Florida, I was searching for the principles that create health.

Just as you cannot reach a destination without fully understanding where you want to go, I realized during my health journey that if I wanted to be healthy I first needed to understand what that meant.

What I discovered, is that health is the result of the consistent application of five timeless principles. By applying these principles, health is guaranteed. Through ignorance of or a failure to apply these principles, disease is assured.

The Preface of this book introduces the many problems of our disease-care medical system. I introduce these failings not to focus on what is wrong but instead to acknowledge the limitations of this system so that together we can then move on to solutions that create health... rather than simply treat disease.

As part of the solution, this book will introduce five timeless principles that create health. In *Timeless Youth* I will show that health is the inevitable end result of the application of these principles and an utter impossibility if they are ignored. It is through the application of these five principles that health, which is a sort of timeless youth, is created.

And with that, let's begin the journey to timeless you[th].

A journey that begins, of course, with you.

# CONTENTS

PREFACE V

INTRODUCTION 1

CHAPTER 1
THE TITANIC PROBLEM 9

CHAPTER 2
THE YELLOWSTONE PRINCIPLE 33

CHAPTER 3
THE MODEL A PRINCIPLE 65

CHAPTER 4
THE QUANTUM PRINCIPLE 91

CHAPTER 5
OLYMPIC STRENGTH PRINCIPLE 115

CHAPTER 6
GOLDEN YOU PRINCIPLE 147

CLOSING THOUGHTS 155

GRATITUDE 157

ABOUT THE AUTHOR 161

SELECTED REFERENCES AND RESOURCES 163

"The farther backward you can look,
the farther forward you can see."

**WINSTON CHURCHILL**

# INTRODUCTION

Dr. Lisa Saunders, a medical doctor, journalist, and professor at the Yale School of Medicine, whose *New York Times* column "Diagnosis" was the inspiration for the TV show *House,* wrote:

"A decade ago, I stood alongside my 99 fellow freshmen as we were welcomed into the ranks of medicine in a 'white coat ceremony.' Here, on our first day of med school, we were presented with the short white coats that proclaimed us part of the mystery and the discipline of medicine. During that ceremony, the dean said something that was repeated throughout my education: half of what we teach you here is wrong – unfortunately, we don't know which half."

That quote, often repeated by the Dean of the Yale School of Medicine, was originally spoken by Charles Sidney Burwell, a past Dean of the Faculty of Medicine at Harvard, over 50 years ago. It is just as true today as when it was first spoken.

This book will explain why half of what is taught in medical school is wrong.

Understanding what is missing in our current disease care system will enable us to create a more complete idea of health. To do so, we would do well to heed the words of Winston Churchill who advised, "The farther backward you can look, the farther forward you can see." So, to best understand the future, we must first look to the past.

Medical school does not begin with the writings of great healers describing what health is. Nor does not begin with great philosophers and their writings on wellness of spirit, mind, and body. Since the question — *What is health?* — is never asked, naturally it is never answered, leaving the path to health shrouded in mystery.

Instead, medical school begins with everything but... including the many names for disease in the body as well as the study of the many parts of the body including anatomy, physiology, biochemistry, and biology. This creates three flaws in our medical system:

1. There is no understanding of what health is. Instead, billions of dollars are spent studying and treating disease while steps to promote health remain hidden.

2. The first principles of health are ignored. Without defining what is health, how are we to know if we are there?

3. Medicine looks at the body as made up of pieces, ignoring the whole (spirit, mind, body) and how the three interact as one.

And despite the research, knowledge, medical technology, and intelligence of the educators, medical education today is deeply flawed. But, please, don't take my word for it.

You may have heard that the word *doctor* means teacher. This is partially true. More exactly, the word doctor comes from the root word *dek* — which means to take or accept. Dek has the same root word as dogma and indoctrination. *Doctor* means to teach, in the sense of to cause others to accept your ideas — to teach in an "I'm right, you're wrong" sort of way. Doctors, in medical school, are indoctrinated into medical thought, a thought process which is wrong 50 percent of the time. Because of this, our whole disease care system is built on a flawed premise.

What if there was a better way? What if, instead of starting with disease and the parts and pieces that make up the body, we started instead with the principles that were true in the beginning and are still true today? This book is about those principles.

To create health, we must find the practitioners who are still applying these foundational principles today. These practitioners are not often found in medical offices or bureaucratic buildings but instead are often hidden in plain sight, diligently applying their craft with patients.

To create health, you must seek not doctors, but healers. While some healers have earned the title of doctor, many have not. Healers may go by many titles including those of chiropractor or naturopath or energy healer or massage therapist or doctor of traditional Chinese medicine or Vedic healers or Reiki practitioners or iridologist, or doula or midwife or functional medicine practitioner or nutritionist or wellness coach or physical therapist or even medical doctor. The title does not matter. What does matter is the result. Healers heal. They do this by making things whole. Whereas *doctor* comes from the root word to take or accept (as in to take or accept the teachings of others), *health* comes from the root word meaning wholeness.

Whereas the disease-focused medical system is based on three flaws, a true health care system would be based on five basic principles:

1. The Yellowstone Principle: The Whole Is Greater Than the Sum of Its Parts

2. The Model A Principle: One Size Does Not Fit All

3. The Quantum Principle: The Power of No-thing

4. The Olympic Strength Principle: How Titanic Problems Lead to Olympic Strength

5. The Golden You Principle: The Power of the Infinite You

How did I discover these principles? Initially, during my two-decade-long journey as a patient in the medical disease care system, and then later, over another decade, as a Doctor of Chiropractic and with a focus on nutrition and holistic healing applying these principles to help patients author their own health journey. And this is where I am today.

If you are wondering about my own personal history, about how my journey progressed toward a healthy and full life, I would start that story by telling you that it began during one of the darkest moments of my life…

It was a Wednesday night, or a Thursday afternoon — but what difference did that make? I lay on my back, in my bed, window blacked out, lights off, door closed. My head propped on a pillow. I tossed and turned for hours, yet, predictably, I could never get comfortable.

I had a headache, but not just any headache. I dealt with "normal" headaches for years. This was not one of those. My head throbbed unrelentingly. To call it a migraine would undersell the experience. My head hurt so badly sleep was a near impossibility. At rest, I felt the blood course through my brain, one painful beat at a time. When I moved, my heart pumped harder and the throbbing in my head increased. When I grimaced in pain, the pounding got worse.

My neck muscles cinched my spine and skull ever closer, including my neck in the agony. To the touch, my neck was stiff and inflamed. I was also nauseous. I hadn't eaten in a day or two. To my right, on my bedside table, perspiration beaded around the now warm glass of water. Despite the thirst, I feared taking even a sip of water as the act of rolling over and reaching for the glass would trigger a new throb of pain from my lower neck to my right temple. A pain so severe it threatened tears. If I didn't move, the pain stayed constant, at a nine out of ten. Any movement shot the pain to an 11 out of 10 — an unbearable level I had borne on and off for 10 years. I actually didn't have to move to make the headache worse. Simply thinking exacerbated the agony. My neck was uncomfortable. My muscles ached.

*Unfortunately, this was the new normal for me.*

*This is how I felt after nine rounds of prescription pain medications. The bottle by my bed said to take every 4-6 hours as needed. When you live in constant, unrelenting pain, what exactly does "as needed" mean? I had taken pain pills every day for the last three years.*

*As I lay in bed, I hoped, I wished, I prayed, as I had for years, for something — anything — to take away the pain.*

*That evening, still in bed, I rolled over and closed my eyes, hoping to wait out the pain. Every time, when the pain was at its worst, I doubted it would ever get better. While the pain never went away, it always improved, usually in two days, three at the most, but at its worst, it was impossible to be sure it would get better this time. When I was mid-headache as the hours ticked by, instead of knowing I was closer to the end, my mind filled with fear, dread, and doubt. What if my headache doesn't get better this time? Shouldn't it already be better? I tried to sleep off the feelings of depression that accompanied the worst of the pain. As I prayed for the pain to go away, the clock ticked by impossibly slow.*

*But this time, rather than give into the depression, I resolved to fight back. For some reason, on this particular day, after a decade of pain, I made a decision. A decision that would forever change my life. I resolved I would not go on living like this — if this could even be called living. For the last decade, normal childhood activities — playing sports, reading, going to the movies with friends, even hanging out with classmates — were largely absent from my life. Outside of school, I saw doctors more often than I saw my friends.*

*Either I would find the solution to my headaches or, I shuddered at the next thought, I would take things into my own hands. I would put an end to the pain, by any means necessary. One way or the other, I resolved, the pain will stop. Even if that meant ending my life.*

*Writing this now, years removed from the pain, it scares me to see those words on paper. I reached a life-or-death sort of desperation. I was determined to solve the problem, one way or the other. With that intention, a journey began.*

"Most of the fundamental ideas of science are essentially simple, and
may, as a rule, be expressed in a language comprehensible to everyone."

**ALBERT EINSTEIN**

# CHAPTER 1
# THE TITANIC
# PROBLEM

On April 10, 1912, the RMS Titanic, with 2,227 passengers and crew,
docked safely in harbor, awaited its first and only transatlantic journey.
At the time, the Titanic was the largest ship ever built, nearly 900
feet long, 25 stories high, and weighing over 46,000 tons. It was the
most technologically advanced ship in the world. Wireless transmitters
that could transmit up to 2,000 miles, farther than any other ship in
existence, were one example of this innovation. A second innovation
was the presence of watertight compartments, subdivisions of the hull
capable of sealing off in the event of an emergency. Even in the worst
possible accident at sea, the builders of the Titanic estimated, the ship
would stay afloat for a minimum of two to three days, allowing plenty
of time to safely rescue all the passengers and crew onboard. And this,
in their estimation, was the worst possible outcome. Because of its size
and innovation, the ship was considered unsinkable. Yet the story of the

Titanic is not a story of technology, innovation, and the biggest ship ever built. It is not the story of a quantum leap forward in maritime transportation.

No, the *Titanic*, as we know, is a story of disaster.

What sunk the *Titanic*? This question has fascinated the public and researchers for over a century. Shortly after its sinking, investigations were launched on both sides of the Atlantic to answer that very question. Throughout the decades since, others have investigated the most famous maritime disaster. We know the *Titanic* struck an iceberg around 11:40 pm on the night of April 14, 1912. The collision ripped a 300-foot gash in the starboard hull. But how did this result in the sinking of the largest, most technologically advanced ship ever built? It was this question that, over 100 years later, we still can't answer. Richard Corfield writes for the Institute of Physics, "No one thing sent the *Titanic* to the bottom of the North Atlantic. Rather, the ship was ensnared by a perfect storm of circumstances that conspired her to her doom."

Let's examine some of the circumstances that contributed to the sinking of an 'unsinkable' ship and over 1,500 deaths:

1. Shortly after the sinking, the *New York Times* quoted a United States official who said the winter weather had produced "an enormously large crop of icebergs."

2. On the night of the disaster, constant north-easterly gales drove ice hundreds of miles farther south than is usually expected that time of year.

3. Astronomers have speculated that the sun and the moon were aligned in such a way that could have led to unusually high tides in January 1912, dislodging icebergs in the Labrador Sea, just southwest of Greenland, and driving them toward

the North Atlantic waters that engulfed the *Titanic* a few months later.

4.  Substandard steel (steel high in pollutants such as sulfur and slag) was used in the construction of the *Titanic* which created a more brittle hull. Upon impact, the more brittle hull ripped instead of bent.

5.  Captain Smith, the renowned captain of the *Titanic*, ignored not one or two but at least seven different warnings of icebergs within 24 hours of the disaster. While other ships heeded the warnings and either slowed down or turned off their engines, the *Titanic* did neither, taking only minimal precautions.

6.  Another theory places blame on the lookouts not having binoculars which were locked up in a storage closet, with the key left in London.

7.  Not only did he not slow down, Captain Smith maintained a speed of 20 knots through the ice field, nearly the *Titanic's* maximum speed, making it harder to avoid the iceberg once spotted.

8.  Evidence suggests a fire may have broken out in a coal boiler room before the *Titanic* left England and remained burning for days during its journey. If so, the fire would have weakened the ship's structure resulting in even more damage from the collision.

9.  The insufficient height of the horizontal watertight compartments, and that the compartments were not watertight vertically, allowed water to spill over the walls into the rest of the ship, exacerbating the damage. As a visual, imagine water in an ice cube tray. Water stays in one compartment until, with enough water, it spills over into the next cube. The watertight

compartments of the *Titanic* were built like this, with walls too short between compartments to contain the water and with no vertical watertight compartment (no lid on the ice cube tray). This meant water in one cube was not contained but instead would overflow into others.

10. Not enough lifeboats. The *Titanic* did not have enough lifeboats for all the passengers and crew making the safe evacuation of all impossible.

Even with all these reasons, our understanding of why the *Titanic* sank and the resulting deaths is incomplete. None of these explanations are sufficient to explain the disaster. Many other ships were crossing the same icy waters, through the same treacherous winter conditions on the same route around the same time and none of them hit an iceberg. Similarly, although there were icebergs in the ocean and the conditions were unusually dangerous, no other ships sank that night. In fact, there had not been a major sinking in the previous 10 years. So, studying the conditions are not enough. To truly understand the cause of the disaster, we have to understand why the *Titanic* was susceptible, and, just as importantly, why the other ships were not.

What caused this tragedy was not any of the 10 reasons listed above. No, the underlying cause was much bigger than this, and much more deadly. Can we blame the lifeboats? How many lifeboats were on the *California* or *Carpathia*, two other ships traveling in similar waters that night? The answer is, who cares? It ultimately didn't matter because they didn't sink. It is obviously prudent to have enough lifeboats, but it is far wiser to never need them in the first place.

Simply stated, what sank the *Titanic* was the belief that it was unsinkable. This single wrong idea directly contributed to each explanation of why the *Titanic* sunk. There was enough room on deck to house lifeboats for all the passengers and crew, but who needs lifeboats on a ship that isn't sinking? Other ships safely navigated the iceberg infested waters that night and all winter either by altering course, slowing their speed or, as the *California* did, heeding warnings and turning off its engines for the evening. However, Captain Smith, describing the *Titanic*, said, "I could not conceive of any vital disaster happening to this vessel... modern shipbuilding has gone beyond that." Overconfidence that no doubt factored into his decision to ignore the iceberg warnings and maintain high speeds through the icy waters. And, with respect to the locked-up binoculars, I have to imagine if there was a real concern about the possibility of the ship sinking, and the subsequent loss of 1,500 passengers and crew, someone would have found some way to unlock the supply closet, right?

On April 10th the *Titanic* was considered unsinkable. By 2:20 am on April 15th, the *Titanic* had sunk.

The Western medical system today parallels the *Titanic* as it sat in Southampton, 111 kilometers southwest of London, days before its journey. The allopathic medical system boasts the biggest hospitals in the world featuring the smartest doctors and the most advanced technology. Allopathy is the name for the conventional medical system, that of treating disease with drugs and surgery. For example, if you have high blood pressure, medicine prescribes a drug to lower your blood pressure. This is allopathy. You identify the symptom or disease and do something that opposes it. Have cancer — radiate it or cut it out. Knee pain — take a pain reliever or have surgery to repair the joint. Allopathy describes a medical system based on eliminating symptoms.

The U.S. medical system is a $3.5 trillion economy — which would make it, if it were its own country, the fourth largest economy in the world. Medical care includes over 4,000 medical and surgical procedures and more than 6,000 FDA-approved drugs. The human genome has been fully mapped and is now used to create specific therapeutic interventions. Add to this virtual reality, robotics, and an exponentially expanding knowledge base of the basic sciences and the medical system is considered the best of the best — almost unquestionably so. As a child, when I had a fever or a headache or a broken bone, neither my parents nor I ever considered going anywhere other than to see our medical doctor. Where else would we go?

And yet, even with the best technology and the brightest minds, in the medical system today disaster lurks in the darkness. Whistle blowers and conscientious observers on the inside warn of this potential disaster. One such voice was Dr. Barbara Starfield, the ultimate insider, a medical doctor, and head of the Department of Health Policy and Management at Johns Hopkins University. In the year 2000, Dr. Starfield published the provocatively titled, "Is US Health Really the Best in the World?" in the *Journal of the American Medical Association* (JAMA). It stated allopathic medical care, (where I had been trained to go since birth) was the third leading cause of death, behind only heart disease and cancer, killing more people than diabetes, influenza, pneumonia, kidney disease, and suicide *combined*. How is it possible that the best doctors trained at the best medical schools as part of the most expensive medical system in the world, kill more people than anything but cancer or heart disease?

Tragically, that is not the worst of the bad news.

In 2006, Dr. Gary Null, an internationally renowned expert in the field of health and nutrition, and his team of MDs and PhDs, reviewed Dr. Starfield's research and found her estimates were wrong — the truth was much worse. According to their research, allopathic medical care kills not a few hundred thousand people a year as Dr. Starfield claimed, but instead between 700,000 and 1,000,000 patients per year — just in the United States. This total number of casualties places medical care as the number one cause of death, killing more people than both cancer and more than heart disease. To arrive at this conclusion, Dr. Null and his team found:

- 199,000 deaths from medical errors in outpatient settings.

- Between 200,000 and 400,000 deaths from the side effects of *correctly* prescribed drugs and medical errors in hospitals.

- 115,000 deaths from the complications due to bedsores during hospital stays.

- 88,000 deaths from infections in medical care facilities.

- 108,000 deaths from malnutrition and dehydration in nursing homes.

- 37,136 deaths from unnecessary surgical procedures.

- 32,000 surgery related deaths.

On the dangers of medicine, two medical insiders both agree the system is deadly. They differ only on the extent of the carnage.

Similarly, many icebergs in the water threaten our allopathic disease care system today, warning us of disaster ahead.

- According to the World Health Organization's (WHO) most recent rankings, released in 2000, the United States health care system ranks 37th in the world.

- Heart disease kills more and more people each year despite incredible advances in open heart surgery, robotics, and diagnostics.

- Despite spending more than half a trillion dollars ($500,000,000,000) on cancer research since President

Richard Nixon declared War on Cancer in 1971, death rates from cancer have hardly changed over the last half century.

- In the United States, we spend more than $3.2 trillion per year, over 20% of our GDP, and almost $1,000 per month for every man, woman, and child in this county, on healthcare. That $1,000 per month exceeds most people's budgets for food, gas, housing, and other common necessities.

- Allopathic disease care is the #1 cause of personal bankruptcy in America.

- Medicare is our government's largest unfunded liability, with a projected deficit three times larger than that of Social Security.

These are the alarms coming over the wireless transmitters, warning us of a *Titanic* disaster. They are the icebergs on the horizon. However, just as the wireless operators on the *Titanic* continued sending out private messages for first class passengers instead of heeding the iceberg warnings from other ships, we are sailing on a sinking ship, ignoring the impending disaster.

The message of this book is that the single most important problem plaguing Western medicine is the dogma of disease care. A malady that sprouts from flawed assumptions and germinates in death and disease. It is this faulty perception that underlies the sinking of the medical system.

What are the false assumptions the system is built on that are sinking medical care? It is the belief in reductionism, studying a single specific and ignoring the whole; it is the belief in a one-size-fits-all approach, ignoring individuality; it is the belief in materialism, that all that matters is matter, ignoring our energetic nature; and the belief that what matters is what can be measured and ignorance of the effects of intangibles, such as stress. It is these false beliefs that explain how the brilliance of doctors, the marvels of medical innovation, and the prolific spending on disease care treatments can result in a system so broken that it is the number one cause of death, greater than even heart disease and cancer. A system so broken that the United States disease care system, which is the epicenter of this idea of heath, ranks lower, according to the World Health Organization, than 36 other countries. The ship of medicine is taking on water.

It is sinking because we are applying a paradigm that is useful in the treatment of disease to try to create health. In an acute health crisis, heroic measures are needed. In those instances, ignoring the principles of health is acceptable, as there is no intention to create health. No one does emergency surgery after a car accident with the intent to promote health. It is done to stave off death. Applying the same principles of heroic medicine that saved a life in an emergency in order to create health will only end in disaster.

But still, despite all its flaws, is medicine really the number one cause of death? When I first heard this, I found it hard to believe. It was hard to believe the second and third time as well — especially with all the knowledge and innovation and research and science and the intelligent, caring people who are part of the system. However, after I spent years going to doctors, taking drugs, undergoing a variety of tests, exploring everything the medical system had to offer and I still suffered in pain now even sicker than when I started, I was forced to accept the medical system was not omnipotent. When I think about why the medical system didn't help me, I think less about what was said in those appointments and more about what was not said. The visits all focused on treating the problem, the disease, with drugs or surgery, but we never talked about how to improve my health.

What is our current idea of health? And how does it compare to what I am proposing? Identifying the current thinking on a subject is hard, somewhat like asking a fish how it likes living in water. To a fish, that is all it knows. It is only when the fish jumps out of the water, and experiences air for the briefest moment, that a comparison is possible.

For me, I grew up living like a fish in the sea of medical dogma and it took years of pain before I ever realized there was another option. This medical dogma of disease care is what underlies the Western medical system — what is called allopathic medicine.

Over the last few decades, a new medical paradigm is emerging, that of functional medicine.

The functional medicine paradigm takes into account the whole body while looking for underlying causes of disease. It uses natural treatments to address these causes. For example, in the case of high blood pressure, functional medicine practitioners might use blood work and other testing to identify the underlying cause of the high blood pressure such as stress, chronic inflammation, or food intolerances and treat these holistically with meditation, dietary changes, supplements, and herbs. Functional medicine is a huge step forward from allopathic medicine, but I would argue we can go even further. This book is about that next step. Because if we don't evolve, I fear our healthcare is setting us up for an epic disaster.

How can this happen? How can researchers tell us that the best doctors practicing with the best technology are the number one cause of death? To understand how this is possible, let me give you an example of a hypothetical patient. Let's call him Joe.

Joe goes to his doctor for a once-a-year "wellness" visit. After Joe's doctor finds Joe's blood pressure is slightly elevated, he is put on a blood pressure medication (ace inhibitor). Six months later, Joe starts taking ibuprofen for an occasional headache. As his blood pressure continues to rise, he adds a second blood pressure medication, this time a beta-blocker. At his next wellness visit he is prescribed a statin medication for his slightly elevated cholesterol level. Joe then develops leg pain, erectile dysfunction and begins to feel sad and lethargic. Joe then is put on an anti-depressant, a drug for erectile dysfunction and his doctor recommends testosterone treatments. What started as a once-a-year wellness visit quickly evolved into more disease and a half dozen prescriptions.

What Joe may not know is that his first medication, the ACE inhibitor, was a gateway drug that led him down a pharmaceutical path of disease care. Headaches are a common side effect of ACE inhibitors. The ibuprofen he takes for the headaches, has side effects which include elevated blood pressure (vicious cycle!) and, well, more headaches. Joe's second blood pressure medication, the beta-blocker, which he needs because of the side effects of the ibuprofen, results in further side effects such as fatigue, erectile dysfunction and, yes, you guessed it, more headaches. Medications for high blood pressure, specifically beta blockers, also cause higher levels of cholesterol. As Joe's cholesterol levels rise, he is prescribed a cholesterol lowering statin drug, a new drug for the side effects of the beta blocker, that causes more fatigue, muscle pain, and weight gain. With this, in the space of just a few short years or less, Joe has gone from someone who was relatively healthy to someone who needs five prescription medications, testosterone treatments, and ibuprofen just to survive.

This is an example of how a focus on symptoms can create more disease. While a blood pressure medication was the first drug in Joe's decline, the actual drug or treatment that causes unintended side effects is different for each of us. Medications are, of course, not bad. In fact, they can be lifesaving, but they always come with side effects. Even when they are lifesaving, drugs are never healthcare. They are disease care. Drugs care for your diseases, they do not care for your health. Unfortunately for Joe, and for all patients like him, side effects are the rule rather than the exception in pharmaceutical disease care.

And Joe's story is not the worst-case scenario. You might know someone like Steve. Steve also went to a doctor for a yearly exam. The doctor did a physical exam, blood work, and a short consultation. The doctor pronounced Steve healthy and asked him to return next year. Days later, while playing with his kids Steve dropped dead of a heart attack. How could the medical system consider Steve "perfectly healthy" just days before he suffered a fatal heart attack? The truth is he wasn't "perfectly healthy." Only a system that doesn't understand health, and instead only focuses on disease care, can confuse being symptom free with being healthy. Steve might have been symptom free, but he was not healthy. And the two terms, symptom free and healthy, are as different as life and death.

With each new side effect, Joe is more likely to be prescribed another drug. With each drug, Joe is more likely to have another side effect. All the while, the concept of health is ignored. With this, the vicious cycle of disease care spins on.

Meanwhile allopathic care sits idle until the patient manifests a diagnosable disease it can treat. As many as 50% of all cardiac deaths occur in patients with no prior history or symptoms of heart disease. In Steve's case, by the time the first symptom presented itself, it was already too late.

Examples like Joe and Steve happen every day. It is because of stories like Joe's that medical care is the number one cause of death — although neither would be counted as a death caused by medicine. In Joe's case, he is still alive, although living with side effects caused by correctly prescribed drugs. And with Steve, he is not counted as a death caused by medicine as his is a death that results from a systemic misunderstanding of what is health.

This is not to say medicine is not heroic and does not save lives. It is, and it does. But even when medicine succeeds, it does so with omnipresent side effects. The problem for Steve and Joe is not in our ability, or inability, to diagnose disease or to create, market, and manufacture new miracle drugs but in our inability to use those tools to create health. Joe isn't sick because he couldn't get the drugs he needed; he is sick because he could. And Steve isn't dead because he didn't visit his doctor for a regular checkup, but because, when he did, his doctor confused symptom free with healthy.

Why is this all happening?

While there are hundreds of differing opinions on what is wrong with the medical system, just as there are many theories on what sunk the *Titanic*, can there be one unifying cause that unites them all?

With the *Titanic*, it was believed to be unsinkable. This false idea, ultimately, is responsible for the disaster.

Is there one underlying cause for our healthcare crisis?

Yes, I believe, there is.

A simple misunderstanding of the word *health* is sinking our current medical system. Rooted in our inability to create health is our difficulty defining it.

Let's start with the textbook definition. The World Health Organization defines health as a "State of complete physical, mental, and social well-being, and not merely the absence of disease or infirmity." This is a great starting point to define health, but it is more of a theoretical definition of health than a practical one. To highlight this point, imagine walking into your doctor's office and asking for help to "improve your mental well-being." If you try this, it is likely your doctor will look at you funny and, if they address your concern at all, may prescribe an antidepressant medication to help with your "mental well-being." Now, some doctors might recommend meditation or prayer to improve your mental well-being, but those are the exceptions and not the rule.

Modern medicine is the best in the world at treating disease. However, while performing a triple bypass is heroic and lifesaving, it is not healthcare. Dr. Denis Burkitt (who discovered Burkitt's lymphoma) once said that raising money to pay for ambulances and a hospital at the base of a cliff is not as smart as building a fence at the top to keep cars from falling off.

Medical care is treating the symptoms of disease. It is raising money for ambulances and building hospitals at the base of a cliff — after the disaster has already happened. Prevention is building a fence. But, even better than that is driving safely, minimizing the need for fences, ambulances, and hospitals.

In the case of the *Titanic*, emergency care is the *Carpathia* steaming full speed ahead to pick up survivors. Early detection might be better monitoring the below water compartments to diagnose leaks more quickly upon impact. But both of those are ways to better treat a problem once it is already present. The optimum, on the other hand, is avoiding the iceberg in the first place. As with the *Titanic* so it is with health — it is far better to create health than to focus on early detection or treatment of a disease that already exists.

Anything else is just rearranging deck chairs on the *Titanic*.

The dominant idea of health is that of allopathic medicine. Although this is often called healthcare, it does not create health and has little to do with care. As I learned during my 15 years as a patient in the medical system and later as a student in Chiropractic school, treating disease follows a simple three-step process:

Step One: Diagnose the problem. As a child when I had a symptom, like a fever and sore throat, my mom would take me to the doctor.

Step Two: Treat the problem. This is often in the form of a drug or surgery to address the cause. With a fever and sore throat, a doctor might recommend Tylenol to lower the fever and prescribe antibiotics to kill the bacteria.

Step Three: Eliminate the symptoms (the sore throat and the fever) by taking the drug.

Within this model of "healthcare," which actually is a system of treating symptoms, what was never asked is why was the symptom there in the first place? Why did I get a sore throat? What caused the fever? Is it too simple to say the fever and sore throat was only caused by bacteria? Were there any factors that might have affected my susceptibility to the bacteria? For example, why did only a handful of my classmates get sick when I did? Or, why didn't my parents get sick while two of my sisters did? Or, how are doctors not always sick when they spend all day taking care of sick people? Clearly, there are other factors than just the presence of bacteria that explain why some people tend to be more susceptible to disease while others stay healthy.

If you have a symptom, the allopathic treatment works to reverse or eliminate that symptom á la Tylenol, antibiotics, or the headache medicines I took as a kid. Allopathy is what is practiced in most every hospital and doctor's office in this country. Every hospital has an *emergency* room, but have you ever been in a hospital that has a *health* room? Not likely because hospitals treat emergencies, not health. Most hospitals organize around diseases, a burn unit, a cancer ward, intensive care unit. Have you ever been to a hospital with a wellness floor? Not likely, because that is not what they do. The medical model of "healthcare" does not promote or restore health, it treats disease.

The implicit promise built into disease care is that if you treat the disease, you will be healthier. Is this true? There are many allopathic treatments that aim to move us away from a disease, but just because we avoid disease does not mean we are getting closer to health.

Treating disease is very different than promoting health. In fact, they are almost opposites.

Taking medications treats diabetes. Eating a diet of whole foods and avoiding refined sugar promotes health.

Anti-depressants treat the symptom of depression. Creating a life of more connection and meaning promotes health.

Statin drugs treat the symptom of elevated cholesterol. Getting optimum amounts of sleep and exercise promotes health.

Drugs treat symptoms. Being healthy eliminates the cause.

There is a fundamental difference between treating symptoms and promoting health.

If we review the health promoting activities above, (whole food diet, avoiding refined sugars, increased exercise, optimum sleep, living a more connected and meaningful life) we will find all of them promote health, and that each activity doesn't just lower your risk of one disease. Each lowers your risk of almost *all* disease. Lowering your consumption of refined sugars decreases your risk of depression and heart disease but also cancer, infection, and diabetes. Living a life of more meaning and connection decreases your risk of heart disease and diabetes. The best part of moving toward health is that, by definition, you are moving away from disease. You cannot be healthy and sick at the same time. The healthier you are, the less sick you will be.

While there are an infinite number of ways to treat disease, we have lost track of the idea that as we get healthier, we reduce our risk for all disease. Because the medical idea of health is an allopathic approach of treating disease, we have a society with more and more diseases, more and more spending on drugs and surgery to treat disease, and less health.

This matters because to create health you don't need to know anything about disease. Instead, to create health you first need to understand what health is — and the principles you must follow. If you use those principles as guideposts on your journey toward health, you can't help but arrive at your destination.

Returning to the *Titanic*, the key to learning from the disaster is, ironically, not studying what went wrong the night of April 14th, 1912, but what was right about the 6,000,000 passenger crossings in the 10 years before, during which just six lives were lost at sea.

Just as patients in countries with older hospitals, less access to the latest drugs, and out-of-date technology are living longer and healthier lives, at lower cost, than patients in the home of the medical model of disease care — the United States — inferior boats in terms of technology, size, and innovation outperformed the *Titanic* in the only metrics that matter, safety, and reliability.

The question is how, and why?

There are five truths that underlie health. These are the first principles, the building blocks, that create healthy bodies, healthy foods, healthy communities and, ultimately, a healthy you. They are:

- The Yellowstone Principle: The Whole Is Greater Than the Sum of Its Parts
- The Model A Principle: One-Size-Does-Not-Fit-All
- The Quantum Principle: The Power of No-thing
- The Olympic Strength Principle: How Titanic Problems Lead to Olympic Strength
- The Golden You Principle: The Power of the Infinite You

A single false belief can undermine great people and great technology and produce disaster. It happened with the *Titanic* a century ago and is happening today in healthcare.

The time has come to examine the idea of health that is creating the current reality.

This book introduces you to a fundamental set of principles that guide health. Principles that are like gravity, invisible yet undeniably obvious in their effects. These principles transcend the prescriptive advice of eat this and don't eat that. In fact, there will be almost no "do this, not that" advice in this book. Instead, my hope is this book will be like a new operating system on a computer — a framework that makes the whole system run better.

The medical system is not broken. Doctors are not bad. Its technology and innovation are not flawed. The medical system, its doctors, and its technology and innovation are all amazing… at treating disease. But, this system isn't designed to build health. Instead, it's killing us.

But the good news is, if we can rid ourselves of our flawed idea of disease and instead upload a new optimum idea of health, we can transform a medical system producing fatal results into one that creates health.

And so my story continues...

*As best I can remember, I was six years old and in first grade when I first experienced a pain in my head. At that moment, for the first time in my life, my head hurt. An initial throb that progressed to a pound. It didn't last long, perhaps just through recess and a bit of the afternoon. I didn't think much of it at the time.*

*With the passage of time, head pain became a more frequent occurrence. When the pain came back, my parents, raised within the medical idea of health, first tried over-the-counter medications to take away the pain. As the headaches continued to progress, I visited my pediatrician. After a few questions and an exam, the pediatrician told us that I had normal childhood headaches. Since the first pills didn't work, he recommended stronger pills. The prescription bottle instructed me to take a pill every 4-6 hours when I had a headache.*

*Over a year later, with the pain continuing to worsen, our family doctor sent me to a neurologist, Dr. Wolfe. He ordered a Computerized Axial Tomography (CAT) scan on my head. Dr. Wolfe explained the test would help him find the cause of my headaches. He was looking for something that was causing the pain, because, of course, headaches had to be caused by some-thing.*

*"We found something on the CT scan."*

*Dr. Wolfe told us the CT scan showed a mass in my head, but it did not clearly show what type of mass it was. The possible explanations for a child with headaches and a mass in his head included a buildup in fluid in the brain, a brain infection, and the dreaded c word, cancer. Each of* which are red flag medical conditions. To find the cause, he ordered a more detailed MRI of my head and rushed me to the front of the line.

After the results came back, Dr. Wolfe had good news. I did not have cancer or an infection or a buildup of fluid in the brain. Instead, I had a cyst in my head that appeared to be benign and possibly had been there since birth. This was the good news. Yet, he explained, even a benign, non-cancerous mass could still cause headaches.

Surgery was the first treatment option to remove the cyst. When he said this, and I thought about someone cutting into my skull to remove something from my brain, you can imagine how I felt. As an eight-year-old boy, I was not scared but instead excited by the possibility of surgery and the idea that there was a thing he could point to as the cause. I was hopeful that finally I had found someone who could give me a reason why I had these headaches. I was raised in the medical idea of health and understood that my headaches were caused by a thing, and I needed to go to doctors to find that thing. The cause, once found, could then be treated with a pill or surgically removed. I reasoned if someone could finally find the thing, then maybe they could do something about it and I could finally get some relief.

Although at first I accepted the idea that a mass might be causing the pain, the more I thought about it, the more I wondered how the doctor knew this cyst was causing my headaches? If, as the doctor said, I was born with a mass in my head, why was I not born with headaches? And how *could headaches that fluctuated in frequency and severity be caused by a mass that didn't change? Some days I had headaches and other days I didn't. Sometimes the headaches were bad and other times they were not. How could this thing, which had been there since birth, be the cause of my symptoms which were constantly changing, often disappearing, and for years never showed up?*

*My journey as a patient in the medical system began not seeking healthcare but instead seeking a treatment for the symptom that had taken over my life. If any of the doctors — pediatricians, neurologists, neurosurgeons, optometrists, orthopedic surgeons, or headache specialists at a world-renowned headache clinic — could have taken away the pain, I would have never left the world of medical care. I hadn't even heard the word chiropractor until days before my first visit and years after my first headache. No one in my immediate or extended family had ever seen a chiropractor, not one. I didn't start on a healthcare crusade; I just wanted my headaches to go away. In an alternate reality, where the medications helped, I would have taken them — faithfully — until I "grew out" of the headaches. And if that day never came, prescription bottles would have been my indispensable lifelong companion. If the pills worked, I might have never understood the difference between being symptom free and truly healthy.*

*But for me, I didn't have that luxury. Circumstance forced me to make a choice, and presented me with a question I was forced to answer: What is health?*

*As a six-year-old, the pain started suddenly. As an eleven-year-old, I had lived in pain for almost half of my life. Severe headaches, the kind that would knock me out for days, came regularly, at least once a month. But these were not the only days my head hurt. I almost always had a headache. In fact, "normal" was how I felt with a headache. Strangely, it felt weird when my head didn't pulse, pound, or throb. At its worst, around age seventeen and eighteen, I had a headache for two years straight. Not pain that was on and off for two years, but one single unrelenting headache that lasted for over 700 days.*

*My headaches, as best I could understand, were an unsolvable, incurable medical condition. Or at least this is what I was led to believe after seeing dozens of doctors over a decade, many, no doubt, with impressive names on their diplomas practicing at prestigious institutions. Despite all their learning, state-of-the-art medical diagnostic tools (MRIs, CT, EEGs, EKGs, visual field tests, nerve conduction tests… the list goes on and on and on) and living in the United States, a country blessed to be on the forefront of medical technology with over $100 billion invested annually in medical research, my headaches didn't improve. Despite following all my doctors' recommendations and navigating the uncertainty when the recommendations of one doctor contradicted those of another doctor, I felt no relief. The best I could hope for, according to my doctors, was that I would grow out of them. After years, I was no closer to* *a solution than when I started. In fact, by any objective measure, I was getting worse.*

*At age seven, back when the headaches began and did not respond to traditional prescription treatments, a neurosurgeon weighed the benefits of brain surgery, to remove a non-cancerous mass in my brain — because maybe, just maybe, that was causing the pain. But even he was not sure it was the cause.*

*Which led me to the question, What do you do when everything you know stops working?*

> "The whole is greater than the sum of its parts."

**ARISTOTLE (384-322 BC)**

---

# CHAPTER 2
# THE YELLOWSTONE PRINCIPLE

## The Whole Is Greater Than
## the Sum of Its Parts

In the early 1990s, conservationists with Yellowstone National Park faced a titanic problem. Over the previous 70 years, an ecosystem that was once in balance was spiraling out of control, and conservationists were at a loss to reverse the trend. One obvious symptom of the change was the ballooning population of elk. But this wasn't the only change. Many of the trees were losing their bark, which led to a decline in the aspens and cottonwoods. Also, the songbird population had decreased. Other changes in the Yellowstone ecosystem included a decrease in the beaver population, erosion of the streams, and a decrease in river animals such as muskrats, ducks, fish, reptiles, and amphibians — many symptoms of a diseased ecosystem.

All the symptoms of change, from beavers to rivers to elk, were connected by a single cause.

The ballooning population of elk led to an overgrazing of tree bark, which led to fewer aspens and cottonwoods, destroying the habitat of the songbirds and providing less wood for beavers to make their dams. Fewer dams resulted in erosion of the streams, and a reduced habitat for muskrats, ducks, fish, reptiles, and amphibians. Naturalists hoped they could attack the problem at its source — the growing elk population.

In the 1930s, the park services started trapping and moving the elk out of the park, and then, when that didn't work, shooting them. This went on for decades. While one symptom improved (the population of elk did decrease) the other symptoms, the trees, birds, and beavers were largely unchanged.

What should be done next? Plant more aspen and cottonwood trees? Introduce more beavers into the park? Dredge the streams and rivers to restore the wildlife habitats? All were logical — capable of treating one symptom or another — but none would restore balance to the ecosystem. Why? Because, as the conservationists learned, the solution to the changes in Yellowstone would only be found by understanding the ecosystem as a whole, and not a disparate set of unconnected symptoms.

While the changes in Yellowstone's landscape were becoming more apparent in the 1990s, the change started in the early 1900s. When the U.S. Park Service took control of Yellowstone from the U.S. Army in 1916, they systematically killed all the wolves in the park, killing all 134 over the next 10 years. From this point until the early 1990s, there were no wolves in Yellowstone as wolves were a deemed a threat to cattle and livestock.

To make the ecosystem whole once again, naturalists could either kill more elk, plant more trees, add fish, feed songbirds, build dams, or, quite simply, they could reintroduce wolves.

Fourteen wolves were reintroduced in 1995 and 17 more the following year. Thirty-one total wolves were added to a 2.2-million-acre national park spanning parts of Wyoming, Montana, and Idaho.

This seemingly small addition produced a series of remarkable changes.

First, the wolves, a natural predator of the elk, helped thin the elk population. Then, the potential threat of being eaten changed the behavior of the elk. The elk moved from the valleys and the gorges, where they could be easily hunted, to the areas of heavy timber. This allowed the bare areas of the valleys and gorges to regenerate. Songbirds and migratory birds returned to the new regenerating trees. The beavers, with their food source of trees restored, began to proliferate. More beavers led to more dams. Otters, muskrats, ducks, and fish that relied on the dams for habitats returned. Increasing vegetation stabilized the riverbanks, reversed the erosion in the riverbeds, and created a healthier ecosystem.

The changes in Yellowstone could not be understood by looking at only one species, one location, or one plant. The interventions aimed at treating a single problem produced only short-lived changes, and none restored health to the whole.

Instead, to restore balance to the ecosystem, all the pieces must be considered as parts of the whole, where every part impacts every other part.

Just as an ecosystem is made up of many individual plants and animals, of a variety of species, each independent yet interconnected, the human body is also made of many independent parts — cells, organs, tissues, and systems, that interconnect to form a whole.

This idea of holism fits within the context of nature. When we introduce wolves back into Yellowstone, we accept the cascade of changes as natural consequences. In nature, we understand that a change to one part affects the whole.

But somehow, along the way, we started to view the body as separate from nature. Instead of seeing the body as a whole ecosystem, the way we might with a national park like Yellowstone, allopathic medicine treats the body as if it operates according to a different set of rules. The body, the thinking goes, is not a whole but instead a collection of parts. This is called reductionism, the idea that a complex system can be understood by understanding the pieces that make it up. It is this thinking that allows us to cut out a cancer from the body without changing the conditions that led it to grow in the first place. Reductionistic thinking let's us take an antibiotic for a cold — often without knowing if the symptoms are even caused by bacteria — instead of asking why the immune system did not fight off the bug in the first place.

In another context, reductionistic thinking allows for the surgical replacement of a knee without evaluating the health of the whole. Specifically, without asking how and why the knee degenerated in the first place. And no, getting older is not a sufficient reason to have a bad knee. My favorite questions for patients who use the "*I'm just getting old, Doc*" explanation for knee pain is to ask, politely of course, "Well, if that is the case, how old is your good knee?"

The idea of reductionism is not universal, but it is foundational to the medical idea of health. Perhaps, it came from the Industrial Revolution with its proliferation of machines to increase output and its concurrent migration into cities and out of nature. Or, perhaps, from the revamping of medical education that occurred after the Flexner Report, in 1910, with its increased focus on scientific research in the basic sciences like physiology and biochemistry (both of which focus on the parts of the body rather than the whole) at the expense of holism. However it happened, the medical idea of health mandates that we see the human body as a collection of parts, separate from nature.

This change had a profound effect on our health.

It is the difference between shooting elk and restoring wolves.

The idea of thinking of the health of the whole is foundational to how we see nature. We do not need to consider the health of 2,000,000+ acres of a national park to see the principle of holism. We can observe the same principle in a single leaf.

When it comes to health, plants are simple. They are not like humans. They don't complain. They don't forget to eat. They don't sabotage their health with Oreos and reality television. They grow. They add carbon dioxide ($CO2$) to sunlight to create food. They survive.

Because of this, healing plants is easy.

A healthy plant needs optimum amounts of three things: sunlight, water, and nutrients (found in healthy soil). A sick plant, one with brown leaves, needs optimal amounts of three things: sunlight, water, and nutrients (found in healthy soil). That's it; that's the whole list. The presence or absence of disease does not change what the plant needs to create health. It may need more or less of each, but healthy plants are the inevitable result of optimal amounts of these three inputs.

But what if things were different? Let's imagine we enter a world of plants, a world that, for simplicity, we'll call Plant World.

Let's imagine Plant World has advanced well past the antiquated ideas of ensuring plants need optimal amounts of sunlight, water, and nutrients. How old fashioned! How antiquated! Instead, in progressive and innovative Plant World, plants are treated like people, following the three-step allopathic model disease care diagnose disease → treat with drug or surgery → eliminate the symptom or disease.

Step one, diagnose disease. In plant world, before a sick plant can be helped, it first needs — of course! — a diagnosis. How can you treat a plant if you don't name the disease? In the allopathic plant disease care, as with humans, the disease is given a name, often with a Greek root. In this case, we'll call it Brown Leafitis. In this progressive system, researchers and plant doctors search for a cure for Brown Leafitis. Lots of money, public and private, is spent researching pharmaceutical treatments and surgical techniques (step two!) to treat the symptoms of Brown Leafitis. The allopathic plant disease care system even has teams of molecular biologists searching for a miracle drug that will cause an already sick plant's leaves to turn from brown back to green. Other promising treatments include, covering the leaves with spray paint and the surgical removal of the brown leaf (a leafectomy, if you will). How progressive! How technologically advanced! Even better, Plant World elected a government that demands equal access for all diseased plants to essential plant medications and includes a team of lobbyists petitioning Plant Congress and the Federal Plant Drug Administration to have medications approved for the new epidemic of Brown Leafitis.

Luckily — for the plants — Plant World disease care doesn't exist. We don't waste our time and money on pharmaceutical drugs or tiny plant surgeries to treat Brown Leafitis. Instead, we restore health in a plant by ensuring the plant has exactly what it needs to create health (sunlight, water, and nutrients (found in healthy soil)). By assuring a plant has the nutrients it needs, the plant returns to health and the symptom of brown leaves go away, or, better yet, never appear in the first place. Giving the plant water, sun, and healthy soil is healthcare. We recognize, intuitively, that a brown leaf is not a disease of the leaf, but rather a sign of a problem within the whole plant. We intuitively provide healthcare to plants. We disastrously provide disease care to humans.

What the medical idea of health seems to forget is that we humans are not reductionistic machines but instead operate under the principle of holism — like plants! In the case of my headaches, taking pain relieving medications sometimes helped with the symptom of head pain, but didn't make me healthier. How could I be healthier taking a chemical that (supposedly) helped pain yet at the same time damaged my liver and kidneys?

Doctors who understood the principles of health would take a different approach. They would see pain in the head not as an isolated symptom but instead as a sign of dysfunction of the whole, much like we view a brown leaf on a plant. Instead of prescribing a drug to treat the symptom, the treatment might include the human equivalent of water, sunlight, and healthy soil needed to restore health.

So how do we find those basic first principles, the human equivalents of water, sunlight, and healthy soil that create health?

We must begin by seeing *a disease of a part* as instead *a dysfunction of the whole.*

Weston A Price, a dentist born in 1870, spent 10 years traveling through five continents in the early 1920s trying to answer the question, "Why do teeth decay?" Dr. Price was motivated by the death of his son from a tooth infection as well as his own personal experience with tooth decay, while eating a "normal" diet. After writing an 1,100-page textbook on dental disease, he had a sobering realization — despite his textbook knowledge of tooth disease, he couldn't answer the question "What makes teeth healthy?" Without this knowledge, he didn't actually know how to make teeth healthy, only how to diagnose, name, treat, and describe them once they were sick.

To find the answer to the question of what makes teeth healthy, he decided to search the world for cultures with the healthiest teeth.

He traveled to isolated islands off the coast of Scotland, the mountains and coastal areas of Peru, the plains of eastern and central Africa, and the islands of the South Pacific, among others. Through his travels he studied the teeth of the native populations who ate their ancestral diet. He found cavities virtually non-existent among these populations. When members of these native populations came in contact with refined and processed foods such as white sugar, white bread, pasteurized milk, and convenience foods filled with extenders and additives, their apparent immunity to dental cavities disappeared proving the cause was not genetic. After they started eating refined foods, their incidence of cavities increased 3,500%!

Upon analysis, he found their ancestral diet contained at least four times the calcium and ten times the fat-soluble vitamins as those consumed by members of the same tribe once they abandoned their traditional diet. Recently, researchers found that ancestral diets have more nutrition than either the diets of the American Heart Association, American Diabetes Association, or the United States government food pyramid. Score one for a diet based on holism.

Price concluded that dental cavities were not a problem of the teeth, but instead were a reflection of the health of the whole. Cavities are but a symptom of a diseased whole. This is the opposite of the reductionistic medical idea of health which says if you have a problem of the tooth, you treat the tooth — fill the cavity, get a root canal, or pull the tooth. While this treats the symptom, it does nothing for the cause, leaving open the possibility of more fillings, more infection, and more dental disease in the future.

So, what was the ancestral diet that prevented cavities and dental disease? There is no one answer to this question. In the Swiss mountains, the ancestral diet consists of high vitamin, raw, unpasteurized dairy products, freshly milled rye bread with meat once per week and vegetables, as available, during the summer. For the native peoples of Alaska, their ancestral diet is dominated by animal sources, with an emphasis on organ meats, and very limited vegetables and seeds. The Australian Aborigines achieved a healthy diet by consuming large and small wild animals, wild plants and, where available, fresh water or marine sea life. The cattle tribes of Africa had a diet that centered on raw dairy, blood, and meat, supplemented by plant foods. The agricultural tribes of Africa ate domestic animals, utilizing their organs, freshwater animal life, insects, and a variety of plants.

There is no magical superfood that connects all five of these cultures, from the agricultural tribes in Africa to the Inuit in Alaska. While we can't discover the one magic food to prevent dental disease, if we look closely, the diets of these cultures, like their dental health, evidence the principle of holism. The healthiest diets of the world are all based on holism. Their foods are local foods and fresh — not refined, fractionated, or filled with additives to extend their shelf life. Since the quantity and quality of nutrients decreases daily between harvest and consumption, with each passing day food becomes less whole.

These cultures developed their ancestral diet, one with 2-10 times the recommended daily allowance (RDA) of vitamins and minerals, hundreds or thousands of years before vitamins were discovered and before the term RDA was coined. They did this with ease because their diet consisted of whole foods. On the other hand, the Standard American Diet (aptly abbreviated SAD) consists of increasing amounts of refined foods, processed foods, and fast foods.

The difference between a whole food and a processed food can be understood by comparing sugar cane and white refined sugar. Sugar cane is a whole food, meaning what we eat matches how we find it unadulterated in nature. Sugar cane, the plant, is filled with B vitamins, over a dozen minerals and is 90% fiber. Table sugar is the processed, refined end product of sugar cane, once the B vitamins, minerals, and fiber are removed. The Standard American Diet (SAD) averages 125-150 pounds of refined sugar consumed per person per year. It is not possible to consume this much refined sugar if you eat the food in its whole food form, as sugarcane. In fact, it would require the consumption of over five pounds of raw sugar cane — per day — to consume an equal amount of refined sugar. To do so, you would have to chew through and spit out hundreds of grams of fiber every day, more than many people taste in a month!

If you did (or even could) eat that much sugarcane, you would naturally be getting an abundance of the vitamins and minerals that are needed to balance blood sugar levels and prevent diabetes. Sugarcane is over 90% fiber which balances the spikes in blood sugar that normally accompany sugar consumption. Sugarcane is high in B vitamins, the vitamins the body needs to utilize sugar, and is also high in zinc, which is needed for insulin production. In short, although sugarcane has some raw sugar, it includes the nutrients needed by the body to process the sugar in a healthy way — mitigating many of the harmful effects of refined sugar. These benefits are lost when sugar is refined.

Fast-food restaurants may be the ultimate example of not-whole foods. While "fast food" in nature might mean grabbing an apple off a tree, today's fast-food restaurants serve foods that are anything but whole. They are loaded with processed ingredients such as trans-fats, refined sugars, preservatives, chemical additives, not to mention genetically modified ingredients and meat laden with hormones and antibiotics. Fast food is so refined, so far from its whole form, that it can hardly be considered food. The use of the term "fast food" is a misuse of the word food. Food does not describe the refined nutrient-depleted menu items served at these restaurants linked to obesity, heart disease, diabetes, and many types of cancer. Food, by definition, is material, usually of plant or animal origin, that contains essential nutrients, such as vitamins and minerals, and is ingested by an organism to produce energy, stimulate growth, and maintain life. It was quite clear that the "fast foods" of today's Standard American Diet (SAD), similar to the refined modern foods Price found in his travels, don't fit that definition. What word describes a food-like substance that causes illness, disease, and death? Poison.

While we increasingly consume our refined and processed poisons at a drive-thru window, or a grocery store, or out of a box, Price wrote about the dangers of refined and processed foods nearly a century ago. The more refined and processed poisons one consumed, the more disease is created — in any part as in the whole. As the individuals Price studied consumed more refined foods, not only did their incidence of cavities increase but so did their rates of infection, heart disease, and obesity.

Sound familiar?

The reason the Standard American Diet is sad is because it consists of refined poisons. The reason the ancestral diet is healthy is because it consists of whole foods.

Despite both ending with the same word, food, there is a vast difference nutritionally between the whole foods and fast foods. Similarly, the terms natural vitamins and synthetic vitamins both share a common word, vitamins, but are worlds apart nutritionally.

I had been taking supplements for 13 years when I saw the headline, *"Vitamin E Supplementation Increases Cancer Risk up to 27%."* I was shocked. I wondered, when antidepressants increase risk of suicide in children, statin drugs cause diabetes, muscle pain and memory problems, and Tylenol sends over 50,000 people to the emergency room each year, how can the mainstream media focus on the supposed dangers of vitamin E? It was the kind of headline I typically dismissed before even reading past the headline.

However, out of curiosity, I clicked on the story to read more. The original article, published in the *American Journal of Respiratory Care and Critical Care Medicine*, read "Long-Term Use of Supplemental Multivitamins, Vitamin C, Vitamin E, and Folate Does Not Reduce the Risk of Lung Cancer." In fact, the study found that not only do supplements not reduce the risk of lung cancer, but they actual *increased* the risk of lung cancer in those who smoke.

*How is this possible?* I wondered. Shouldn't those who smoke benefit most from vitamins?

In school, I was taught smoking damages the lungs by speeding up the production of free radicals. Free radicals are molecules that injure the body and contribute to a variety of diseases including cancer. Free radicals are created as the result of normal body processes, like the production of energy in the cell as well as from environmental toxins such as those from smoking. That is the bad news. The good news is there are helpful molecules called antioxidants, like vitamin E, that can neutralize free radicals. So, I thought, vitamin E should decrease the risk of death from smoking related cancers — not increase it.

To understand how a free radical causes damage in the body, imagine a small dance, one with four couples in which each dancer has a partner. Then, a single partnerless dancer arrives, taking the total number of dancers from eight to nine. The odd dancer out, the free radical, does not have a partner and can only dance by cutting in on one of the existing couples.

In the body, when the free radical cuts in, it breaks up an existing structure, such as DNA, cell membranes, or the lining of arteries, resulting in disease. Free radicals are linked to the development and progression of many diseases, from aging to cancer to Alzheimer's and heart disease.

Antioxidants, such as vitamin E used in the study, work by bringing an extra partner to the dance, taking the total number of dancers from nine to 10. Now the free radical, previously roaming the dance floor, cutting in and disrupting the other pairs, has a partner. Now each couple can dance uninterrupted. Because antioxidants limit this damage, they must be good.

The article continued "Fruits and vegetables are associated with a lower incidence of lung cancer." This statement reinforced my idea that consumption of foods high in antioxidants vitamin C and E, like fruits and vegetables, lower the risk of lung cancer. The cancer protective benefits of fruits and vegetables have been proven again and again, showing that people who eat the highest amounts of fruits and vegetables, naturally high in antioxidants like vitamin C and E, have the lowest risk of cancer. Yet here we find the difference. How do antioxidants in fruits and vegetables decrease cancer risk while antioxidants in supplements increase the cancer risk?

The answer is that not all antioxidants are created equal.

Antioxidants can be generalized in two primary groups, those that are made by nature and those that are made by humans. Natural antioxidants are found in foods, especially fruits and vegetables. The body also makes natural antioxidants, as well. Synthetic antioxidants are those made by humans in a laboratory. These are found in almost all supplements.

What I was not taught in school is that free radicals are more than just the evil byproducts of energy production in the body; free radicals are also necessary for life. You can die without free radicals. For example, natural free radicals are produced by the immune system to kill pathogens like bacteria and, as it turns out, cancer. The immune system uses free radicals, the partnerless dancers, to "cut in" on pathogens and cancer cells to stop their growth. While it is true that free radicals "cutting in" in the wrong place can be bad, it is also true that when they cut in under the right circumstances they can be very helpful. Free radicals are both essential for life and potentially dangerous. They, like the wolves added to Yellowstone, can both kill and heal.

The immune system uses free radicals to kill cancer cells. Those who took the highest amount of supplemental vitamin E, in the form of a synthetic antioxidant made by humans, had the highest risk of lung cancer. The more human-made antioxidant supplements someone took, the higher their risk of lung cancer. This correlation was strongest in those who had smoked the longest. This means that the more someone smoked, the more they were affected by synthetic vitamin E. Because free radicals are used by the immune system to kill cancer, synthetic supplements were neutralizing the body's own cancer-killing free radicals. This is less of a problem in non-smokers as they are much less likely to develop cancer in the body. However, once the cancer cells are present, the body needs its immune system to hunt and kill the rogue cells. Only then, with cancer cells present and the immune system compromised by synthetic antioxidants, are the dangers of the synthetic supplements especially problematic.

The study didn't show antioxidants caused cancer. Instead, it showed that antioxidants allowed cancer to grow more quickly in those who already had cancer cells present as it impaired normal immune cells.

But this pro-cancer effect was only found in synthetic antioxidants.

To understand the difference between the dangers of synthetic antioxidants and the benefits of fruits and vegetables, we have to understand the difference between antioxidants made by nature and those made in laboratories. Vitamin E is defined by the National Institute of Health (NIH) as alpha-tocopherol, a single chemical that is a potent antioxidant. And yet there is just one problem: alpha-tocopherol is not vitamin E, at least not according to nature, which has the audacity to disagree with the NIH.

In nature, vitamins are never found as isolated parts. It is impossible to find alpha-tocopherol by itself in nature. Impossible. Following the fallacy of reductionism, the medical idea of health defines vitamin E as alpha-tocopherol. When vitamin E is found in nature, it does contain alpha-tocopherol but alpha-tocopherol is also found with delta-, gamma- and beta-tocopherols, as well as essential fats, nutrients, and minerals such as selenium that are part of the vitamin E complex. No food has alpha-tocopherol without the other components of the vitamin E complex. In short, in nature, alpha-tocopherol is always part of a team.

Another difference between supplements and foods is natural sources of the vitamin E complex are made by plants from soil and sunlight. In contrast, synthetic alpha tocopherol, as found in supplements, is often made from petroleum. Imagine drinking petroleum and expecting that to be good for your health.

The headline didn't say that taking supplements made from petroleum increased the risk of lung cancer. If it had, one could easliy accept the results of the study. You don't need to be a doctor to know drinking petroleum does not promote health.

Does vitamin E promote cancer? The answer to that question depends on if we use the term "vitamin E" to mean man made vitamin E, or the whole vitamin E complex as found in nature. Synthetic vitamin E, as the research showed, does increase the risk of cancer in smokers, yet those with the highest consumption of fruits and vegetables, thus consuming the whole vitamin E complex, had the lowest rates of cancer and disease.

Holism heals and reductionism kills. This is as true of vitamins as it is of food.

Research on the dangers of synthetic supplements is not new. According to nutritional pioneer Dr. Royal Lee, nutrition scientist Dr. Agnes Fay Morgan of the University of California, Berkeley showed dogs fed diets enriched with synthetic vitamins died more quickly than those fed food without added vitamins. That has never been disproved. Dr. Morgan did that in 1942, just when companies began adding synthetic vitamins to food. Foods enriched with synthetic vitamins will kill animals quicker than unenriched foods.

Close to a century later, the Yellowstone principle still has not been accepted as true. Vitamin supplements are often still made from synthetic isolated ingredients that are marketed as being as beneficial as eating whole foods rich with natural vitamin and mineral complexes.

So, while the average health-conscious consumer hears the headline and concludes that vitamin E causes cancer, the underlying truth is synthetic vitamin E in supplements is not the same as the whole vitamin E complex found in nature. Reductionism mistakes a single compound for a whole. When we apply the philosophy of reductionism to vitamins, we find synthetic antioxidants made from petroleum increase cancer risk. When we apply the principle of holism, we find foods rich in vitamin and mineral complexes reduce the risk of cancer.

When you introduce wolves into Yellowstone, trees grow, birds return, and balance is restored. Yet, when you "treat" the overpopulation of elk with reductionistic intervention, like hunters, you get the worst of both worlds — unintended side effects and a system still out of balance.

The allopathic medical system is built on reductionism — measuring parts, diagnosing parts, and treating parts. Parts, parts, parts! The best medical researchers are those who become experts on a single part of the body, or even better, a single type of cell in a single part of the body, or even better a single reaction in that single cell type in that single part of the body. In short, the best researchers are those who know more and more about less and less.

Like researchers, the most respected and highest paid doctors are the ones who are the most specialized. The medical system validates, rewards, and promotes reductionistic thinking every step of the way. It is a foundational principle of the medical idea of health. General practitioners, doctors who deal with the whole body, are one of the least popular concentrations in medical school (the more specialized the better!). A general practitioner is less respected than an oncologist, who is, in turn, less respected than a pediatric oncologist who, in turn, is less respected than a pediatric oncologist specializing in leukemia. The simple rule for doctors and researchers to increase their standing in the medical system, and their pay, is specialize, specialize, specialize.

This is not to say specialization is without benefit. The medical system is the best in the world at understanding the structure and function of our smallest parts. Yet, if we study the parts without understanding the whole, we risk failure — like the story of six blind men and the elephant.

There were once six blind men who stood by the roadside every day, and begged from the people who passed. They had often heard of elephants, but they had never seen one; for, being blind, how could they?

One morning an elephant was driven down the road where they stood. When they were told that the great beast was before them, they asked the driver to let him stop so that they might see him.

Of course, they could not see him with their eyes, but they thought that by touching him they could learn just what kind of animal he was.

The first one happened to put his hand on the elephant's side. "Well, well!" he said. "Now I know all about this beast. He is exactly like a wall."

The second felt only of the elephant's tusk. "My brother," he said, "you are mistaken. He is not at all like a wall. He is round and smooth and sharp. He is more like a spear than anything else."

The third happened to take hold of the elephant's trunk. "Both of you are wrong," he said. "Anybody who knows anything can see that this elephant is like a snake."

The fourth reached out his arms and grasped one of the elephant's legs. "Oh, how blind you are!" he said. "It is very plain to me that he is round and tall like a tree."

The fifth was a very tall man, and he chanced to take hold of the elephant's ear. "The blindest man ought to know that this beast is not like any of the things that you name," he said. "He is exactly like a huge fan."

The sixth was very blind indeed, and it was some time before he could find the elephant at all. At last, he seized the animal's tail. "Oh, foolish fellows!" he cried. "You surely have lost your senses. This elephant is not like a wall, or a spear, or a snake, or a tree; neither is he like a fan. But any man with a particle of sense can see that he is exactly like a rope."

With too much focus on parts, we risk, like the six blind men, losing sight of the whole.

Blood work helps doctors understand the tiny cells of the blood, counting their contents bit by bit; CTs and MRIs visualize the anatomy of the body; vision tests measure the acuity of the eye. Each test visualizes and quantifies a piece of the whole. Because of these advances, doctors can diagnose disease earlier and more exactly and administer treatments down to the cellular level. This can be, and is, tremendously valuable (and impressive!) but it is not health.

Reductionist tests are tools, but without seeing the whole you risk missing the big picture, just as you cannot understand the ecosystem of Yellowstone by examining a single piece of bark.

In 1999, I went to a chiropractor to get rid of my headaches. As I described the pain in my head, this healer didn't limit his evaluation to just my head. Instead, through muscle testing, he evaluated the health of the whole and prescribed treatments that had little to do with the pain in my head. He advised me to change my diet, take two supplements, and with this, I left the office.

What I discovered over the course of working with him, is the pain in my head was like the dying aspens. It was a symptom of a problem, yes, but it was not the cause.

Hippocrates, a contemporary of Socrates and Plato, said, "It is more important to know what sort of person has a disease than to know what sort of disease a person has." That is holism. Because the allopathic medical system is designed to look at a patient, a condition, a symptom, and a problem reductively, we treat the symptoms of high blood pressure, cancer, heart disease, and obesity separately—even when they occur in the same person.

Lisa, a 46-year-old woman, had been a patient in my office for over five years. She had battled with psoriasis, an autoimmune condition marked by red, itchy, scaly patches of skin, for over three years. She also had pain in multiple joints earning her the additional diagnosis of psoriatic arthritis. The condition started after a period of heavy stress, when she discovered her boyfriend of many years was cheating on her. This hit her hard, as it would anyone. She was a working single mother with two teenage boys. She had a full plate before managing the stress of a breakup and uncovering a web of lies and infidelity. To add to this, she now had a new health challenge — an autoimmune condition — to manage. By following a modified autoimmune disease diet (she strictly avoided soy, milk, wheat, and sugar), and supporting her body with whole food supplements, she was able to better manage the symptoms. She was improving. Then, after a year of sustained progress, the psoriasis flared up again. This time worse than her initial symptoms. A pattern of flare ups interspersed with periods of improvements is common with psoriasis. At first, I treated her the way I had before, using diet and nutrition. But this time was different. She wasn't making progress like before. At best she was treading water. *What changed?*

I thought more about her story, looking for the underlying cause affecting the whole. For six months, we evaluated her for immune challenges, chemical toxicity, heavy metals, and food and environmental allergens that could be triggering her symptoms.

For six months, we failed to find the underlying cause.

One Monday afternoon, Lisa was the last patient of the day, arriving at 5:30 pm. Her eyes showed a bit of redness and evidence of swelling and, as soon as I said hi, she brought her hand to her face to wipe away a tear.

I lowered my voice to ask, "What's going on?"

"It's nothing," she said.

I invited her to sit down. "Stressful week?" I asked.

"Like you wouldn't believe."

She went on to tell me about the stress of full-time employment as a medical assistant, a part-time business as a freelancer, the stresses of being a single mother, and, at the very end, she mentioned that she suspected her current boyfriend was cheating on her. She told me she had suspected this for a while but had recently found more clues. She felt sure her suspicions were correct. As she told me the story, she started to cry, again. I handed her a tissue.

"Was there a moment of shock?"

"Yes," she said with a laugh. As if to say, isn't that obvious?

This may not be a question that is typically asked in a medical office and I think that is exactly the problem. I believe one of the reasons the medical system is failing is because we are ignoring the whole person. Shooting elk didn't work in Yellowstone and pretending that the stresses in a patient's life, whether they be connected to work or relationships or family, don't affect their health doesn't work either. According to the CDC and medical textbooks, 60-80% of all disease and doctor visits are caused by stress. And yet, on how many visits is stress addressed?

The skeptics might say, who can be sure? Who has found the biochemical mechanism that connects a cheating boyfriend to psoriasis of the skin?

That is exactly the point. Even the question belies a reductionistic bias.

Who has found the exact mechanism connecting the loss of wolves to river erosion? If we are looking for clear A causes B then we would deduce, that wolves do not effect river erosion. But health, like Yellowstone, is not reductionistic. It is more butterfly effect — a phenomenon whereby a small change in one location, like a butterfly flapping its wings in Rio de Janeiro, can have an outside effect elsewhere, as in changing the weather in Chicago.

What if instead of looking for a direct cause and effect relationship, we step back and look at the big picture. Then there are many possible connections between stress and psoriasis. The truth of the interconnected wholeness of us as humans has been noted for millennia, going back at least to Plato, 2,400 years ago. This sentiment was echoed by Dr. William Osler, a Canadian physician who practiced in the late 1800s and into the early 1900s. Dr. Osler is a legend in the field of medicine. He is one of the four founding professors of Johns Hopkins Hospital in Baltimore. He created the first residence program for specialty training of physicians (the emphasis of specialization runs deep!). For all his accomplishments he earned the title The Father of Modern Medicine. In 1892, he wrote that rheumatoid arthritis (of which psoriasis arthritis is a subset) has "in all probability, a nervous origin." He noted "the association of the disease with shock, worry, and grief." Saying, essentially, that the health of a part is a reflection of the health of the whole. Today, the National Psoriasis Foundation notes that psoriasis is associated with serious health conditions including depression. But these ideas don't fit into our current model of disease care. However, just because they don't fit in our understanding of the world, doesn't mean they are not true.

I wanted to probe the shock Lisa identified for a connection. A shock is a moment of collapse. A moment when one's dreams and goals in an area suddenly crash. It is a time one feels small and crushed by the circumstances of life. As you read this definition, an example of a shock in your own life might come to view. In the body, the painful emotions of a shock can manifest in a variety of ways. I asked Lisa a specific series of questions about the shock, reasoning that the most important thing I could do as a doctor, for her physical health, was address the emotional pain she was sitting in.

As I went through the questions, the most notable emotion was frustration. As she tapped into that mood, the tears returned until something almost magical happened. After asking her questions to work through the frustration, she went from feeling upset and stuck in the emotion of the experience to feeling empowered about her ability to choose how she responded.

She reconnected to her dream of a happy loving relationship that crashed at the moment of the betrayal. As she experienced the negative and reconnected to her dream, an amazing thing happened. The shock she was stuck in released. Her mood lightened and she was more here, in the present moment.

Even more inspiring, she smiled.

I gave her homework to journal further about the shock. She gave me a hug and thanked me as she left.

Eight weeks later, she returned to the office. I glanced at the paperwork she filled out in the office and saw she reported that her symptoms of psoriasis, the itching and blotchy redness, had improved. She even noted significant improvement in other symptoms such as joint pain in her hands and her headaches.

"What happened?" I asked.

In addition to continuing to experience the frustration instead of running from it, she found conclusive proof her now-ex-boyfriend was cheating on her. She confronted him and kicked him out of the house. Her stress level dropped considerably, and her smile returned.

Lisa was back, and so was her health.

So, what does your relationship with your significant other have to do with the health of your skin?

Looking at it through the reductionistic medical view of health, we see psoriasis, a disorder of the skin, as a skin issue. It is treated most commonly with topical corticosteroids, a medication applied to the skin which reduces inflammation and swelling. While these help treat the symptoms, by making the skin less red and itchy, they don't handle the underlying cause of the redness, swelling, and inflammation.

I could have given Lisa something to treat her symptoms, even something natural like a supplement or natural therapy, but it would not have created health. Health of the body is a reflection of the health of the whole, including spirit, mind, and emotions.

We will explore this idea more in future chapters in the Model A Principle and the Olympic Strength Principle, but for now what is clear is we cannot create health by only treating a part. Health comes from the root word for wholeness and to create health we must consider the whole spirit, mind, and body.

One of the great shortcomings of the reductionist assumption of health, is that it sees an individual as a series of parts. Have an issue with your heart, go see your cardiologist. Have an issue with your spouse, go see a psychologist. If your blood sugar level is too high, go visit an endocrinologist.

In my own journey, I visited a pediatrician, general practitioner, neurologist, neurosurgeon, orthopedic surgeon, orthopedist, massage therapist, hematologist, and an optometrist, among others. Each saw me as a piece of a whole — a sick body, a brain, a nervous system, bones, joints and muscles, eyes, biochemistry etc. And yet, the health of the whole can never be understood examining only a single piece — no matter what that piece may be. Just like none of the blind men understood the whole of an elephant by only touching one part.

What constitutes a whole, as I would come to find out, extends beyond the body. Holism, the same principle that helped us understand the healthiest diets and the healthiest supplements, also applies to people, spirit, mind, and body.

Louis Pasteur is a well-known name in science. He was a French chemist and microbiologist who pioneered discoveries in the principles of vaccines and pasteurization and helped eradicate diseases such as diphtheria and typhus. He is a big deal. Less well known is his contemporary, Claude Bernard, who insisted, in opposition to Pasteur, that it was not so much the presence or absence of microbes such as bacteria and viruses that caused infection, but rather the health of the organism that determined its susceptibility to disease. In other words, the health of the whole was more important than the presence of a pathogen. Whereas Pasteur would focus on the bacteria or virus that causes the disease, Bernard would say the health of the organism was more important than the microbe as it determined their susceptibility to disease. The healthier someone is, the more resistant they are to microbes in the environment. The two contemporaries were at odds for years, Pasteur promoting germ theory of disease claiming microbes caused disease, and Bernard arguing that it was not the pathogen that mattered but the health of the whole. The healthier the organism, Bernard would argue, the less the pathogen matters.

This debate was finally settled when Pasteur apparently gave up on his own theory just before his death. Pasteur's dying words were reported to have been, "Bernard was right. The microbe is nothing, the terrain, everything."

By analogy, imagine a patch of grass with weeds growing in it. Pasteur would say the weeds are the problem. Bernard, on the other hand, would say the problem is the grass is not healthy, as the weeds are only there because the lawn had bare spots which allowed the weeds to grow. In this example, Pasture would focus on killing the weeds while Bernard would focus instead on planting seeds to create a healthier and fuller lawn. If a lawn is green and healthy, Bernard would argue, it won't have weeds — there would be no room for them to grow. It is when the lawn gets sparce, where there are patches of dirt without grass, that weeds grow. Pasteur warned about the dangers of weeds. Bernard would say weeds are a sign of a sick lawn. Make the lawn healthy, he argued, and you won't have to worry about weeds. Although the medical idea of disease adopted Pasteur's germ theory and marginalized Bernard's theory of the whole, Pasteur on his death bed acknowledged Bernard was right, it is the health of the whole that matters.

This is holism.

As I ventured on my own journey of healing, this was a surprising realization. However, maybe it shouldn't have been, as the word health comes from the German root kalio — meaning whole.

Health, quite literally, sprouts from the roots of wholeness.

And here's where I'll pick up my story...

*When I was 11 years old, just 18 months before the headache I wrote about earlier, I went to a world-renowned headache institute. It was a fancy sort of place, long wait times for appointments, impressive diplomas hung on its walls, doctors pioneering research.*

*My family and I were desperate to find anything to help. My headaches continued to get worse. One day we decided to go to the best. This institute was the nation's first comprehensive head pain treatment and research center. It was described as the Mayo Clinic for headaches. And it was within driving distance from our home.*

*The three-hour initial appointment included blood work, a physical examination, a neurological examination, a consultation with two different doctors and a nurse, more bloodwork and an extensive health history. After the first appointment, I was invited to return for a second visit to review the findings.*

*Two weeks later, as the doctor walked into the room, I was impatient, nervous, and optimistic that the internationally renowned center with its multidisciplinary teams would finally be able to offer relief.*

*As the lights flickered, the doctor told my mom and me, that the headaches I had were of the migraine variant variety. As opposed to traditional migraines, tension headaches and cluster headaches which each follow a typical presentation, migraine variants were the fourth, catch-all category of headaches — symptoms variable, cause unknown.*

*My eyes lowered to the floor.*

*My mom leaned over to put her hand on my shoulder, to see how I took the news.*

*I wanted to cry.*

*Another dead end?*

*Why did I have to have the kind of headaches that even these doctors didn't know the cause of?*

*I assumed this meant that they would not be able to treat the headaches.*

*However, the doctor had some good news for me. He explained that his team designed a treatment program specifically for me. The roller coaster of hope, after free falling, started to rise again. I would start on a low-dose antidepressant, 5 mg of Elavil which I was told was not being prescribed for depression but as a headache preventative and a stronger medication, a muscle relaxer, which I would take every day.*

*This combination of medications offered hope, the doctor assured us.*

*"But what about the other pain killers I'm taking?" I asked.*

*The doctor explained that, in their experience, there was a fifth type of headache — a rebound headache. This headache is caused by the overuse of pain medications. Since my pediatrician four years ago told me to take a 500 mg Ibuprofen every four to six hours when I had a headache, and since I had a headache almost every*

4-6 hours during those four years, I had taken a lot of Ibuprofen. Nearly the maximum dose every day — for years. The doctor explained my body had developed a chemical dependency on the drug and explained the drug was poisoning and destroying my liver.

The best treatment for breaking the rebound cycle was to stop the use of pain killers. This may, the doctor cautioned, intensify the pain at first but then lead to improvement later. If there was one thing I could bear, it was pain. The short-term pain would be easy to bear if it gave me hope of breaking the rebound cycle.

"So the doctor thinks my headaches are caused from taking too much prescription medication. Right?" I asked my mom during the drive home.

"Yes."

"And that is why he stopped the one medication I was taking and put me on two more?"

"Yes," she responded.

"How does that make sense?"

Even without understanding the how or why, my mom and I trusted the doctor and I started on the program he recommended. I took the medications and followed their instructions — thinking it was my only hope. When the doubts crept in, I reminded myself that these were some of the best doctors in the world, with impressive diplomas and all the rest. But also, I came to the sad realization that there was nowhere else for me to turn. This had to help, *because if it didn't, I didn't know where I would go next.*

*My mom picked up the medications from the pharmacy and set the pills next to me at dinner.*

*"Do you want me to get you some water to take this?"*

*"No, I got it."*

*Pop. Swallow. Done.*

"I desired to know why one person was ailing and his associate,
eating at the same table, working in the same shop,
at the same bench, was not."

**D. D. PALMER**

---

# CHAPTER 3
# THE MODEL A PRINCIPLE

## One Size Does Not Fit All

Outside Detroit, in the early 1900s, was a factory that would revolutionize the automotive industry. It began as a 60-acre facility, considered the largest factory in the world when built, and over the next 15 years grew even further to include an additional 2,000 acres. Supplying this complex required over 700,000 acres of forest, iron mines, and limestone quarries in Michigan, Minnesota, and Wisconsin, coal rich land in Kentucky, West Virginia, and Pennsylvania as well as a rubber plantation in Brazil. The transport of all these raw materials required a dedicated fleet of ore freighters and an entire regional railroad. It was a titanic operation.

As a result of the innovation and sheer size of this complex, the once-niche automobile boomed in popularity. In 1899, 30 American automobile manufacturers produced a combined total of 2,500 cars. In 1923, this one factory alone rolled out over 1,800,000 automobiles.

The automobile was the Model T.

The company was the Ford Motor Company.

Also in 1923, blocks away from Ford, a competing car company named a new CEO. At the time, this competitor, General Motors, owned just 12% of the car market, a distant second to the dominant Ford. Alfred Sloan, the new CEO of General Motors (GM), announced GM's new policy: A "car for every purse and purpose." This policy was a direct shot at Ford and the Model T. At the time, Ford's factory produced only one type of car, the Model T, with no optional equipment or upgrades. Ford offered one type of payment — in full at purchase. Every Model T customer paid the same way, for the same car, painted the same color, black.

For a while, this was a huge success. Ford sold over 15 million Model Ts during its 20-year run. Henry Ford, the founder of Ford, derided those who encouraged him to listen to customer feedback. Ford reportedly said, "If I had asked people what they wanted, they would have said a faster horse." Sloan, on the other hand, dared to question the status quo. He made it a point to talk to customers, dealers, and salespeople to find out directly what the customer wanted. With his "car for every purse and purpose" policy, Sloan envisioned a company that offered customers different models with different options, and, gasp, even different colors. At the time, it must have seemed crazy to question the most successful car ever built, manufactured in the world's largest factory, by the number one automobile manufacturer in the world, but that is exactly what Sloan and GM did.

In 1921, Ford sold two-thirds of all the automobiles built in the United States — every one was an identical black Model T. By 1926, three out of every four cars were purchased using financing — none of which were black Model Ts. The very next year, in 1927, the final Model T rolled off the production line, and with it, the innovative but hyper-specialized Ford assembly line screeched to a halt. After years of resisting change, Ford finally had to accept the reality that individual customers had individual needs and wants. Ford was forced to replace the one-size-fits-all Model T with the individualized Model A. Car buyers are not Model Ts. Ford was forced to recognize that people are not one-size-fits-all machines.

Medicine today makes the same mistake as Ford in the 1920s. It assumes patients are much like the Model T itself — all the same color, same shape, and built of the same parts. Since one-size-fits-all doesn't work for something as simple as a rain poncho (when is the last time you put on a rain poncho and thought, wow, this fits great?), how can we expect it to work for something as complex as the human body with its 30-40 trillion cells?

Much as Ford increased production by stamping out individuality and manufacturing a one-size-fits-all product, the medical factories of today, the hospitals and doctors' offices around the world, are increasingly becoming an assembly line of sorts — increasing throughput by streamlining visits and limiting the doctor-patient interaction. Yet unlike the days of Ford, this assembly line is not increasing the affordability of its product. In fact, medical care has never been more expensive. Medical care gives all the impersonality of assembly line manufacturing without any of the economic benefits. It is the worst of both worlds.

Just as the future of the automobile industry in the 1920s lay in recognizing the individuality of the customer and offering them choice, so too does the future of healthcare lie in recognizing the individuality of each patient and in the offering of unique solutions that reflect this individuality.

There exists a man who, in spite of drinking almost a liter of Scotch whisky every day of his adult life, lived until he was 93. He managed a successful business until just before he died. We all know someone like this, right? Well, maybe not someone who drinks that much Scotch, but maybe someone who ignores the most obvious of health recommendations, who smokes or never exercises or eats a plate of bacon per day but lives healthfully into old age. These people are easy to hate. They are the people who can sit on the back porch and smoke, while we slave away in the gym, and yet still appear healthy. These are the ones who make us scream that life is not fair.

What makes this Scotch drinker unique is that he was studied by researchers who wondered, how could this man drink so much alcohol and yet appear so healthy? Based on what is regarded as "normal," this man should have been sick, grossly deficient in many nutrients with severely diseased organs. He should have never made it to his 60s. Instead, he was in excellent health, productive, active, and coherent even into his 90s. Let's call this the curious case of the Scotch whiskey man.

There exists a different sort of person, this one a close relative, who eats a very clean diet. Her diet is plant based with the occasional serving of fish, largely organic, fresh, and prepared at home. She is a yoga teacher, a physical therapist, has a body that exudes fitness, and takes whole food supplements to support an already exemplary diet. Her cheat food is a brown rice cake. And yet, health challenges continually, well, challenge her. Low energy, fatigue, constant headaches, bloating, hormonal issues, and digestive distress are all a daily part of life. As a teenager, she qualified and competed in the Boston Marathon, but that was the past. Despite following healthy habits for over a decade, she hasn't been able to run more than a few miles without feeling ill. Call it the curious case of the My-cheat-food-is-a-brown-rice-cake yoga teacher.

The idea that there is a standard set of nutrient requirements for all humans, or a single ideal diet, is flat out wrong. It isn't true. This idea has been disproven again and again in the literature, and over and over again in my practice. Yet, this research is probably unnecessary as most of us know someone like the curious case of the Scotch whisky man as well as someone like the My-cheat-food-is-a-brown-rice-cake yoga teacher. What gives?

We are each individuals. Scientists, speaking scientifically, call this biochemical individuality. This term was popularized by Roger Williams in the 1960s. Roger Williams, a preeminent scientist and professor at the University of Texas Austin, had a leading role in the discovery of three different B vitamins. He knew a thing or two about nutrition. And of all the things he knew about, of all the wisdom he wanted to share, he most frequently and fervently shared one single message: that we are all unique. One size does not fit all. He literally wrote the book on biochemical individually called, incidentally enough, *Biochemical Individuality.* He shares the curious case of the Scotch Whisky Man in this book. Just as Ford's Model T went extinct because he ignored the individual wants of his customers while others listened, Williams warned against doing the same in the field of medicine. Most nutrition, Williams derided, is based on statistically average humans.

"Nutrition is for real people," Williams said. "Statistical humans are of little interest."

To understand Williams' problem with "statistical humans," imagine two groups of individuals. The first group, which, for convenience, we will call Group 1, consists of 10 men. All are roughly the same height, have average amounts of muscle and fat, average fitness, average amounts of hair, an average tendency to consume alcohol, average sized feet, average emotional reactions, and average eyesight. They all work in similarly average jobs and are from average economic backgrounds. In brief, all are similarly average.

The second group, let's call this one Group 2, is also a group of 10, although it consists of both men and women. Within this group, one is quite muscular, one more obese, one with exceptional endurance, one bald, one an alcoholic, one who is quite tall, one subject to fits of anger, one pregnant, one a factory worker, and one who is nearsighted.

You take a statistical average of Group 1 and offer them a one-size-fits-all rain poncho, and, you know what? Because they are pretty much the same, the poncho may kind of fit. And yet, in Group 2, each individual is so different the average is worthless. The one-size-fits-all poncho won't fit any individual in Group 2 well. In fact, the individuals in Group 2 are so different from each other, can we even assume they all would want a poncho? We are quick to prescribe a one-size-fits-all solution without even considering if one may prefer an umbrella or even walking (and possibly singing) in the rain.

It is much easier to develop one-size-fits-all recommendations for Group 1. For doctors, the more similar their patients, the more they can assume about them, their life, their diet, their stresses, and their wants, and the quicker they can diagnose problems and prescribe a solution with mass-production-like efficiency. The more you assume the statistical average person researchers use to represent all humans, the more you assume we live in a Group 1 world. Just as important, the stronger researchers and doctors hold to that assumption, the faster the assembly line can run. Group 1 thinking facilitates assembly line medicine. Because once you have seen one black Model T, you have pretty much seen them all.

Almost every book, study, research paper, and article assumes on some level we are a standard Group 1 sort of species. The slight problem is that we do not live in a Group 1 world. The assumption we live in a Group 1 world is a generalization of convenience, yet one without truth.

Individual variation is the rule not the exception. We have dozens of shoe sizes. Some of us have no hair. We humans exhibit wide varieties in height, skin tones, levels of stress, toxin exposures, and muscle tone. Nutritionally, Williams found nutrient requirements can vary four, 20, even 100 times from person to person. While 16 glasses of Scotch per day is a recipe for disaster (nutritional and otherwise) for *almost* everyone, some rare souls don't evidence signs of deficiency and disease. Williams found our nutrient requirements are unique, as unique as we are. Yet, the medical idea of health is stuck diagnosing disease with assembly line level efficiency while it prescribes a one-size-fits-all solution.

Where does the individuality we see in humans, the very individuality that makes us a Group 2 species, come from? To try to answer this question, scientists peered into our genes. Genes are parts of DNA and are encoded in a relatively simple language. Despite its simplicity, (it consists of only four letters, A, T, C and G), DNA has the ability to encode incredible individuality through its sheer volume. The genome has approximately three billion gene pairs that reside within 23 chromosomes, present in each and every cell of the body. And, like a fingerprint, each individual's genome is uniquely theirs.

The very foundation upon which biology is built holds that one section of DNA, a gene, is transcribed into ribonucleic acid (RNA) and then translated into a single protein. This belief is so widely held, so unquestioned in its acceptance, it is not referred to as a theory but as the central dogma of biology. (Imagine that — dogma, a word most commonly used to describe matters of faith, here being used to name a foundational principle in science!) This dogma describes a one-way flow of information, from the DNA of genes into RNA and then into protein. In a way, it proposes a model of genes that, like Ford's Model T, lacked customization, as the one-way flow of information meant the genes we are born with are ours forever.

Doctors hoped that by understanding the genes we were born with, they could then predict future medical conditions allowing medicine to treat disease before it even showed up. At least that was the hope. The first step toward this possibility required a fully mapped human genome. In 1990, the Human Genome Project set out to do just that. This project became the largest collaborative biological project in history and included the work of teams of researchers all around the world.

Just as a basketball player might warm up for a game by first practicing layups, global researchers began the process of mapping the human genome by first mapping the genome of much smaller organisms — the fruit fly and roundworm. They found the common fruit fly had 13,000 genes and a 1-millimeter roundworm had a slightly larger genome of 18,000 genes.

Since scientists knew there were 70,000-90,000 proteins in the human body, they expected humans to have at least that number of genes according to the one gene = one protein central dogma of biology. After allowing for a few extra genes — instructing where the code for one protein ends and the next begins, scientists settled on the expectation of roughly 100,000 genes in the human genome. Researchers reasoned this number made sense as the 30-40 trillion cell human body is orders of magnitude larger and more complex than the fruit fly and the roundworm.

However, researchers didn't find 100,000 genes.

Not even close.

Instead, scientists found that the human genome, fully sequenced in 2003, contained only 25,000 genes.

What happened to the 75,000 missing genes?

The question of the missing genes turned the central dogma of biology on its head. Scientists wondered; how could we make all the necessary proteins from only 25,000 genes?

Professionally, researchers and scientists were baffled by the results. As humans, they may have been humiliated, genetically speaking, to be only slightly more complex than a fruit fly or a roundworm. The results couldn't be right.

Only they were. Once it was confirmed that yes, in fact, this was correct, scientists turned their attention to understanding how it was possible. Scientists reasoned humans must have a way to customize a genome that was previously thought to be fixed. We must add increasing variation to a surprisingly simple genome. To explain how this was possible, the field of epigenetics was born.

Epigenetics is the field of genetic communication. It explains how our body gets feedback from our environment, our diet, and our choices to customize the expression of the genome. Just like Sloan listened to customers, salespeople, and employees before building a car tailored to their needs, epigenetics listens to signals from the environment to customize the expression of our genes.

The word epigenetics is a combination of the prefix epi- meaning above or upon and the word genetics referring to our genes. This gives epigenetics a literal meaning of above or beyond the genes, as in the factors that control our genes lie outside the genes. Practically, this means factors such as nutrition, exercise, levels of stress, and the environment all influence how genes are expressed. Epigenetics explains the individualized expression of our genetic code.

To illustrate the principle of epigenetics, imagine a rather large bookcase full of books, 25,000, in this case, in which each book represents a single gene. Ninety-nine percent of the genome of all humans is the same. Said another way, 99% of the books on each of our bookshelves are the same. Based on this fact, we should be a Group 1 sort of people. But we're not. Instead, scientists now recognize that while we may share 99% of our genome with the rest of the human population, we each express that genome in our own unique way. Just because we all have almost exactly the same books on the shelves, does not mean we would all start reading the same book. It turns out, if you start in the middle of one book and stop in the middle of the next, you are likely to get a different story than reading any one book by itself. For example, if you read the beginning of a biography of Plato and the end of *Goodnight Moon*, the resulting story will be very different than reading either book on its own. Epigenetics, then, is the science of how our choices, lifestyle, and environment individualize the expression of our genes. In fact, through epigenetic mechanisms, one gene can be expressed in up to 3,000 different ways. This allows for the needed complexity to turn 25,000 genes into over 70,000 proteins. In short, epigenetics explains the individuality of genes that the central dogma of biology ignores.

The vast differences we observe from person to person, from hair color, to height, to metabolic rate, to liver function, the very things that make us a Group 2 sort of people, come from the 1% of our genome that is different and the individualized expression of that shared 99%.

Yet, the central dogma of biology and the medical idea of health hold that our genes determine our health. And if this central dogma of biology were true, the idea of one-size-fits-all medicine makes a bit of sense because if we are our genes, and our genes are 99% the same, then, more or less, we are all the same. We would be a Group 1 sort of people.

On the other hand, epigenetics argues that our choices, lifestyle, and environment all individualize the expression of our genes and these factors are more important than our genes. Epigenetics tells us we are not 99% the same but 100% unique. And this uniqueness has profound implications for our health.

If genes were a one-size-fits-all prescription of health (and disease), identical twins would have identical health outcomes. Yet, researchers have found the lifespan of identical twins vary widely, with an *average* gap of more than 15 years. In twins with 100% identical genes, lifespan varies greatly. Our health destiny, it turns out, is not written into our genes. Instead, it is found in the library of life. Epigenetics tells us we have the power to choose the books we read and how we read them. The addition of this choice means we are not one-size-fits-all machines but rather as unique as our individualized environment.

In my office, like in the medical factories, I ask each patient for their family history of disease, but I don't confuse the idea of family history of disease with a genetic history of disease. They are not the same thing. To prove this, researchers have studied what happens to adopted children in their new families. It turns out, the adopted children often develop the same diseases as their adopted family. Yet these children don't share genes with their adopted family. So what explains this connection?

Family histories of disease still matter, but not because of genetics. Instead, it's because we inherit a lot more from our family than just our genes. From our family members we often learn, consciously or unconsciously, what to eat, how to eat, the importance (or unimportance) of exercise, what sorts of careers are acceptable (which affects things like stress levels and toxin exposures) and which are unacceptable, how to handle (or not handle) stress, how to communicate (or not communicate) our feelings, among many other behaviors.

For most diseases like heart disease, cancer, and obesity, genetic factors account for only 3-5% of all cases. While there are some purely genetic diseases, such as Down Syndrome in which patients have a third copy of the 21$^{st}$ chromosome, diseases like this are the exception not the rule. Most diseases, instead, are like heart disease, cancer, and obesity, in that they have genetic risk factors but are not genetic diseases.

While genes contribute about 3-5% to our risk of disease, all other factors combine to explain the other 95-97%. While genes offer a one-size-fits-all explanation of disease, they are as obsolete as the Ford factory after the death of the Model T.

The benefits of individualization over one-size-fits-all solutions are evident at least as soon as baby's first meal. It has been said that breast milk is nature's perfect food, an ideal combination of protein, fat, carbohydrates, vitamins, and minerals. This is true, but what makes it perfect is more than just the nutrients it contains but also in the individualized way a mother provides them to her baby. Breast milk constantly changes its nutrient contents, exactly as the needs of the baby change.

A baby's first meal from a mother's breast is called colostrum. This thick golden milk supplies an easily digestible meal to the newborn. In comparison to breast milk, colostrum is lower in fat and lactose and higher in carbohydrates, protein, and potassium to support the immediate needs of the newborn. It also provides the newborn their first immunity boost as it is rich in infection fighting IgA molecules. At the same time, colostrum is rich in probiotics supplying the nutrients needed to colonize the infant's microbiome. Breast milk is, above all, dynamic, changing like Sloan's automobiles according to the exact needs of the newborn.

As amazing as this is, the individualization does not end here. Not only does breast milk change over time, but it is individualized in response to a whole host of factors, including gender, as breast milk for boys contains 25% more calories than it does for girls. It is individualized based on the feeding stage, as the first milk a baby consumes during any given feeding, called foremilk, is packed with more carbohydrates, protein, and vitamins as well as a higher water composition to protect the baby from dehydration while the hindmilk, produced at the end of each feeding, is thicker and darker in color, with increased energy and fat content. It is individualized based on time of day as evening breast milk contains more sleep-inducing hormones. If the child is sick, breast milk will contain more infection fighting antibodies. Because of this this, mother's milk can start treating the baby for a disease long before it is ever diagnosed by the doctor. Breast milk is even individualized based on the weather as the warmer the temperature, the more water breast milk contains to prevent dehydration in the child. Nature's perfect food is perfect because it is individualized to the exact needs of the child.

Even more amazing, if the mother has twins, the breast milk each baby suckles will be unique. There exist feedback mechanisms between mother and baby which allow Mom to tune into the individual needs of her child and give each child a customized food tailored to their exact needs.

It is the incredible individualization of breast milk that makes it nature's perfect food.

In the 1960s, doctors attempted to re-create breast milk in a lab. Its components were measured, quantified, and combined. The assembly line was built. The only problem was, it didn't work. Formula-fed infants were at an increased risk for many health problems including cancer. Furthermore, mothers who didn't breast feed also suffered from an increased risk of breast cancer and it took them longer to lose the baby weight. Scientists and doctors alike learned the static synthetic replication of mother's milk was not an effective substitute. Mother and baby both suffered. Why? Not only did they ignore individualization, they lost track of the whole. Imagine trying to recreate Yellowstone by first counting all the creatures and plants and fish and streams and then tossing them haphazardly anywhere. It wouldn't work. The magic of Yellowstone is not found in the number of trees and plants and birds and animals but instead in the incredible synergy created between them. Similarly, the magic of breast milk is not found in its parts but in the synergistic function of the whole. Infant formulas violate both the Yellowstone Principle as well as the Model A Principle of health.

If nature's perfect food changes in response to the individual needs of the baby, as well as its environment, time of day, and weather, how then can we then assume there is a single, one-size-fits-all diet that works for us adults? Are we not making the same mistake as the formula-promoting doctors and scientists of the 1960s? As it turns out, we are.

The nutrition label grades each food's nutrient content against generic nutritional recommendations. It is based on the mythical average person needing a 2,000-calorie diet and the false assumption we live in a Group 1 world.

The nutrition label has roots going back to 1941, when the Food and Nutrition Board established the original Recommended Dietary Allowances (RDAs), to prevent disease in both soldiers and civilians during World War II. The original RDAs set guidelines for calories and eight essential nutrients.

When the RDAs were established, they were created to prevent disease during wartime. RDAs were never about creating health. They were about disease prevention. This is a crucial distinction as the level of a nutrient that prevents disease is vastly different than that which creates health. Consider a nutrient like calcium, the minimum amount that prevents a disease like osteoporosis is very different than the amount that creates optimally strong bones. Just because a patient doesn't have osteoporosis doesn't mean they have optimal bone health. Even today, you could drive a century-year-old Model T to get you from Chicago and New York. But, with a top speed of 40-45 miles per hour, no air conditioning, no shock absorbers and (gasp!) no phone charger, it is not going to be an easy journey. Just because it will get you there, does not mean it will be optimal, With nutrition, an RDA that prevents disease is only a start on the journey of health. Nutrient levels that prevent disease are not the same as those that promote optimal health, just as a Model T will get you there, eventually, but it will be a much tougher trip.

A second issue is that the RDAs of today ignore individuality. Originally, in the 1940s, the RDA of a nutrient for an individual depended on three factors: age, sex, and parity (are you pregnant?), recognizing at least some individual variation among nutritional needs. Over time, these differences blended into the universal nutritional recommendations we find on the label today. In the ultimate of ironies, representing a gut punch to Dr. Williams' legacy, we now have a one-size-fits all RDA for 29 different nutrients, including the B vitamin Williams first isolated and named (folic acid B9) and the two others he helped discover (B5 and B6). Today, RDAs are calculated to be sufficient to avoid disease for 97.5% of the population. This means that even if we consume the RDA of a particular nutrient, one out of every 40 people will still be deficient in that nutrient. Not only do the RDAs not create optimal health for anyone, for some they don't even prevent disease.

Is there any proof that we change from having individualized nutrient requirements as a newborn to label-ready uniform nutritional needs as an adult? No, not only has one-size-fits-all not been proven in human nutrition — remember even the original disease preventing RDAs reflected *some* individuality — there is incredible evidence in favor of individualized nutrient requirements. In fact, there has never been a nutrient — vitamin, mineral, or otherwise — that didn't show marked individuality.

The assumption in nutrition is there is a statistically normal human, that humans are a species of Group 1 people, and that this statistically average Group 1 person needs a statistically average quantity of vitamins, the same as all the other similarly average humans. It's the idea we all are the same black Model T with universal requirements for gasoline and motor oil. We are told our nutritional needs are all the same, or at least close enough for government work. This is decidedly not true.

A few examples of known individuality in nutrition include:

- Weightlifters need more protein.
- Endurance athletes need more B vitamins.
- Menstruating women need more iron.
- Sugar junkies need more zinc and B vitamins.
- Infection increases our need for zinc, vitamin C, calcium, vitamin A, and essential fatty acids.
- Stress increases our need for minerals such as calcium, potassium, magnesium, and manganese as well as B and C vitamins.
- Pregnant women need more of everything.

Humans are dynamic beings. None of this is reflected in the one-size-fits-all nutrition labels. Just as the nutrient requirements of a newborn are dynamic and constantly changing, so are the nutrient requirements of adults.

The principle of individuality does not only apply to the nutritional needs of the body but also applies to its anatomy. We find incredible variation throughout the body. The sciatic nerve travels through the muscles of the buttock in one of 13 different configurations. Depending on this configuration, some are more prone to back pain while others escape this predilection. Some stomachs can hold as much as eight times more than others. Individual taste thresholds vary up to 20x, explaining some people's love for spicy foods while others tear up just thinking about it.

If we look closer at the heart, there are many examples of anatomical variation within this one organ.

- The shape of the right atrium, one of the four chambers of the heart, has over 12 different variations in shape and valve placement.

- In a study of healthy young men, heart rates ranged 233% from 45 to 105 beats per minute.

- The same study found the heart's pumping capacity varied in healthy young men, up to 342% from 3.16 to 10.81 liters of blood per minute.

- In the aorta, the main artery leaving the heart, there are at least six different possible configurations of the aorta and its main vessels — just in its first two inches.

- Also, the size of the aorta can vary by a factor of three.

Variation in size and shape of the heart is so common in childhood that the typical average heart, according to researchers, is rarely seen. The idea of an average is a myth, like a well-fitting poncho. These are not just interesting facts. Life and death decisions are made each day based on one-size-fits-all idea of a normal heart. Doctors use these "normals" to determine when patients need cardiovascular treatments and even when they need heart surgery. Researchers in Vienna concluded using "normals" that don't recognize anatomical differences owing to gender, age, height, and weight means some patients are getting drugs they don't need, and others are not getting the drugs they do. Even worse, some people are getting heart surgery they don't need, and others are not getting the surgeries they desperately do need. Ignoring individuality is not only failing to treat disease, but through side effects of drugs and surgeries, it is creating even more disease. We are a Group 2 sort of people, and this is evident in our nutrient requirements, our genetic expression, and even our anatomy.

Trisha came into the office with a story all too similar to my own. She first had headaches in 1993 (two years after my headaches began) as a 25-year-old working for a large real estate brokerage. As her headaches got worse, they started interfering with her work and life. She began searching the medical world for help and tried, in her words, "every migraine drug that existed" including antidepressants, muscle relaxers, and Hydrocodone, an opioid based pain reliever. She went from doctor to doctor, drug to drug. This went on for years, but the headaches did not improve. Eventually a neurologist noticed an alarming find on her MRI. He saw a part of the cerebellum being pushed down through the base of the skull. He announced he had found the cause of her headaches. *Finally,* she thought. The neurologist gave her the diagnosis of a Chiari malformation. To visualize what a Chiari malformation is, imagine trying to shove a square peg through a round hole only, in this case, your brain is the peg and your skull is the hole. A Chiari malformation is a structural defect in which the cerebellum is pushed down through an opening at the bottom of the skull. The neurological complications of this compression include headaches and neck pain.

With the Chiari malformation visualized, her doctor announced he had found the problem. They had proof on the MRI. Trisha trusted her doctor. After years of trying drugs for an unknown cause, she now had a cause she could see. *This was progress*, she thought. The medical treatment of a Chiari malformation is brain surgery Specifically, a surgical procedure in which the hole at the bottom of the skull is opened wider and a piece of the neck bone is cut out. If you make the round hole bigger, and create more space, this will take the pressure off the brain and the symptoms will subside — or at least that was the hope.

Trisha followed the doctor's advice and had the surgery to repair the Chiari malformation. The surgery was a success, at least according to the doctors. Unfortunately, Trisha didn't consider the surgery successful. After the surgery, she woke up in worse pain than she had before. "It should get better over the next few days," the doctors said. It didn't. Trisha felt disheartened and depressed. Her post-surgical rehab included months of painful physical therapy — all this on top of the financial cost of surgery. She still had headaches only now they were worse than before. Because of pain, she was forced to quit her job. Years later, she took a trip to the Mayo Clinic where the doctors told her she should not have had surgery (*No shit,* Trisha told me was her thought upon hearing their conclusion). At Mayo, she was prescribed more pain meds and biofeedback therapy. Over the next decade, her headaches continued to worsen. Working continued to be a struggle on good days and impossible on bad days. She felt maxed out doing part-time work babysitting a child. When she finally made it into my office, she told me, she had suffered from daily headaches for over two decades.

I was reminded of my own story, as multiple doctors told me the cyst I have in my brain was the cause of my headaches. However, unlike Trisha, the doctors advised my parents and I against brain surgery. As I grew older, from a seven-year-old boy into my teen years, I struggled with the doctor's explanation that the cyst was the cause of my headaches especially when repeated MRIs showed the cyst was not changing while the pain in my head constantly changed.

Trisha's story was the counterpoint to my own. She had headaches that multiple doctors said were caused by an MRI finding. She got the surgery, had the "cause" removed, and still had the pain. As she told me her story, I thought about the two rules I use to apply the Model A principle: one, anything can cause anything, and two, every effect has a cause. The trick is to find out what that cause is.

In Trisha's case, we identified a series of possible causes of her headaches. An individualized nutritional examination revealed a sensitivity to refined sugar, wheat, and dairy products. In addition to this, we used a series of nutritional supplements to support the health of her body, including her thyroid, kidneys, and immune system. On top of this, I was curious if there were any stressors in her life that might contribute to her symptoms. I asked Trisha what was going on in her life 25 years ago just before the headaches first began. She remembered a relationship that had ended just around that time. It was a relationship that brought up tears and the scars of emotional abuse. Scars that were still raw a quarter century later. Knowing this, we treated her as an individual — an individualized dietary program, an individualized program to handle the specific underlying emotional stressors that preceded the first headaches, as well as specific chiropractic adjustments to help her body heal.

As of the time of writing, Trisha has been a patient for over five years. At her last visit, Trisha told me she had only one headache in the last seven weeks, after veering from her prescribed diet with a barbecue dinner. This was the longest she has gone without a headache in decades. She reports a 90% decrease in headaches since she started care, after years of progressively worsening pain. We have not solved every health issue she has, but her life has been transformed by the near absence of the symptom that dominated her life for twenty-five years. A transformation made possible by recognizing her individuality.

After the death of the Model T, the factory that once produced over 5,000 cars per day had to be shut down for almost five months. In the end, Ford learned their lesson, ignoring the individual was accelerating its own destruction. One-size-fits-all often meant one-size-fits-none and was on its way to bankrupting the company.

Incorporating these lessons, the future of Ford was such a radical departure from its past that the old monolith of a factory was now obsolete. Over 40,000 tools had to be thrown out. Months later, after the retooled factory reopened, Ford introduced the Model A as their answer to the successes of General Motors and the death of the one-size-fits-all Model T. The new Model A, replete with options and choice, bore a closer resemblance to the automobiles of Sloan's General Motors than to the Ford's Model T. Customers embraced the Ford Model A, because Ford embraced the individual.

And so my story, my search for answers and relief from the relentless pain, continues…

*Five years later, my mom, dad, three sisters and I, gathered at my grandparents' house. I remember it was Christmas Eve and as we enjoyed an Italian Christmas complete with stuffed shells and fried mozzarella, my grandfather pulled my father aside.*

*"How are Jeffrey's headaches?" my grandfather asked, already knowing the answer.*

*I sat alone after carrying my food to a quiet corner. The headache was mild, but I was still in pain. Within a few hours, I would go into a bedroom to escape the Christmas music and holiday lights and try to sleep off the pain. I overheard their conversation from half a room away.*

*"Remember last year we talked about the doctor in Atlanta? I really think you should go," my grandfather said. My grandfather stood nearly six feet tall, with Sicilian heritage and a commanding jaw. When he spoke, people listened.*

*He continued telling my dad, "Your mother and I talked to Evelyn again last week and she is still doing well."*

*Evelyn was a friend of my grandparents who lived in South Carolina. She had bad headaches, suffered with them for years — like me — had seen many doctors who couldn't help her — like me! — until she finally went to an alternative doctor in Atlanta and now her headaches were much better, even gone.*

*I leaned forward, setting down the food. The pain softened.*

*My grandfather continued, "Michelle is a freshman in Atlanta, I'm going to visit her in a March. Why don't you have Jeffery meet me there?" It was less a question more a command. "Yes" was the answer.*

*So that's how, shortly after my 14th birthday, in March of 1999, I ended up in Atlanta visiting my cousin Michelle at college and then lying on my back in the office of an alternative doctor — a chiropractor who specialized in nutrition.*

*We arrived on a Friday morning and drove directly to the office. The office was unlike any I had ever been to. It was a small yellow building, a converted house that looked like it was built in the 1920s. It was far from the impressive buildings of traditional medicine I was used to.*

*"Are you sure this is it?" my mom asked me as the taxi pulled in.*

*"Yes, I . . .I think so." The address on the paper matched the numbers on the building, but the building hardly matched my idea of where I thought I was going.*

*After finishing the initial consultation, (which consisted of a 30-minute case history — with just one doctor!), I lay down and experienced muscle testing for the first time. No blood work, no neurological testing.*

*As I would learn later, muscle testing is when a practitioner uses an indicator muscle such as the deltoid of the shoulder to test a system of points corresponding to organs and muscles. So imagine this, I am lying on my back and the doctor pushed my arm with one arm while touching a series of points with the other. Sometimes, my arm stayed strong and other times my arm went weak. Based on the points where my arm stayed strong and where it went weak, the doctor formulated his opinion.*

*It was weird. I laughed. Not inside, not quietly, but openly, with the doctor about a foot away.*

*This is nuts! I flew all the way here for this?*

*I couldn't understand what he was doing.*

*I would later learn muscle testing is based on the principles of acupuncture and traditional Chinese medicine and recognizes that integrity and balance in the energy flow of the body is vital for health. By testing specific contact points, the practitioner can gain great insight into the function of the body.*

*At the time, none of this meant anything to me.*

*As the visit ended, Dr. Marc explained that he found evidence of heart and digestive stress and that I should take two supplements, one to help with each.*

*While the exam and evaluation were, to say the least, way out there, the idea of taking a pill was very familiar.*

*It is what he said next that really confounded me.*

*"I want you to cut out sugar and dairy from your diet."*

*"What do you mean?" I asked with a look of surprise.*

*"I don't want you to eat any refined sugar or dairy, no*

*cookies, cake, soda, milk, cheese, yogurt, ice cream…"*

*He continued to talk but I was lost.*

*"What's left?" was all I could ask in response.*

*Months later, when I went back for the second visit, I stopped laughing and started asking questions.*

*"How have your headaches been?" the doctor asked.*

*"I'm not sure I understand how, but I think I do feel better."*

*He smiled.*

*While I wasn't healed, not by a long shot, I wasn't worse. For the first time in years, I visited a doctor, followed their instructions, and the headaches were not getting worse. This was a major, major win. In fact, I thought I was even feeling better. The idea of healing was so foreign to me, I hesitated to believe it was possible. I had not once visited a doctor in seven years and had my headaches get better.*

*To me, this small win was a miracle, the first signs of progress. At the end of the visit I wondered How does all of this work?*

*I struggled to understand how food supplements and energy testing could help me feel better as I was educated and raised in the medical idea of drugs and surgery. And this was a long way from that thinking!*

*How does all this work? The search to answer that simple question sent me on the journey of a lifetime.*

"If there is any ultimate stuff of the universe, it is pure energy...
subatomic particles are not 'made of' energy, they are energy."

**GARY ZUKAV *DANCING WU LI MASTERS***

---

# CHAPTER 4
# THE QUANTUM PRINCIPLE

## The Power of No-thing

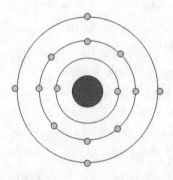

When I was in fifth grade, my teacher, Mrs. Stanczyk taught my classmates and me about the atom. The atom, she explained, was the building block of the universe. Our science textbook showed a simple model of the atom, one with the nucleus at the center surrounded by electrons which circle the nucleus. Mrs. Stanczyk assigned my classmates and me a project, to make a model of the atom. I used spare change to make my atom, gluing nickels and dimes together to represent the protons and neutrons of the nucleus and pennies to wire circling the nucleus to represent the electrons. What my rudimentary model of the atom showed was an atom that was made of things — tiny little things.

In my model, it was coins which represented the particles that make up the atom. Science books teach that the building "blocks" of the universe are atoms and that the building "blocks" of the atom are smaller protons, neutrons, and electrons. And because atoms form molecules which form the cells, tissues, and organs of the body, the human body is also made of things. The medical idea of health follows the thinking of my fifth-grade textbook, that we live in a world made of things.

But is this true? For millennia, scientists and thinkers assumed the universe was made of small particles, tiny Legos that combined to build the cosmos. This is widely assumed but never proven. In fact, even today, scientists refer to what I learned in my fifth-grade textbook as *atomic theory* — never rising to the level of atomic fact. Why? Because even with all the amazing advancements in science, no one has ever seen an atom. Without proof, the best scientists can do is assume.

What I never learned in school was that if the model of atom I made in fifth grade was scaled correctly, with dimes and nickels glued together to represent the protons and neutrons of the nucleus, the closest electron on my model should not have been just inches away glued to wire, but instead should have been over a mile away. The truth is that atoms are over 99.996% space — something the science textbook, and the models of my classmates and I, woefully misrepresented.

Even though the atom is 99.996% space, it's not exactly empty. What quantum physics, the evolution of physics championed by Einstein among others, teaches us is that "empty" space is actually not empty — it is full of energy. Energy then, not the atom, it is the true building block of our universe.

$$E = mc^2$$

Ultimately, the atom is made of energy, which means, of course, that you and I and the cosmos are made of energy. Einstein's famous equation, E = mc², says the energy of an object (E) is equal to the mass of an object (m) times the speed of light squared (c²). Often this is understood as Einstein saying mass can be converted to energy and that energy can be converted to mass. While this is true, the truth of the equation runs much deeper. With a simple equal sign (=) in the most famous equation in physics, Einstein is communicating that *mass is energy* and that *energy is mass,* erasing any distinction between the two. Applied to health, this means our body, which we often think of as a real thing made of mass, is ultimately made of energy.

Einstein's simple equation, and the equal sign between the energy and mass, revolutionized physicists' understanding of the universe. The quantum revolution would go on to change the understanding of the motion of planets, light, and gravity. It would lead to breakthroughs in the fields of semiconductors, superconductors, and computers. It led to the first coherent theory of chemistry. But most importantly, it revolutionized the atom and taught us we do not live in a universe of things.

With medical care, the dogma of disease care is based on a preoccupation with things and an ignorance of energy. When a stone falls into water, the water ripples. Ripples in the water are the visible effects of waves of energy traveling through the water. Many times, disease in the body is like ripples in water. We observe the disease in the body, like ripples, but the cause, the first pebble to fall, begins energetically. Let's consider the example of heart attacks. To prevent heart attacks, doctors look for a marker of heart disease. The medical system focuses on things as causes. The most common thing medicine uses to predict heart disease is cholesterol. Blood work can measure cholesterol. Drugs can treat cholesterol — and effectively at that. Yet we know that 50% of patients who have heart attacks have normal levels of cholesterol. Studies have even shown patients with higher levels of cholesterol, a molecule vilified for its role clogging arteries, have *lower* rates of heart attacks than those with the recommended levels of cholesterol. Despite cholesterol monitoring and treatment, incidents of heart disease continue to increase year after year. So, the treatment controls the symptom, the thing, but not the problem. Cholesterol is a ripple in water, it is an observable manifestation but not the cause. Lowering cholesterol by itself does not create health.

So, what if we looked for a cause of heart attacks that went beyond things? One potential cause of heart attacks is stress. Stress is not a tangible thing. As such, it is often ignored in the medical system. What we do know is sudden stressors, such as the death of a loved one, can spike the risk of death from a heart attack 1,800%. A sudden loss, while not a tangible thing, triggers a stress response in the body, which is a very real event. A sudden loss is the stone that falls in the water. An 1,800% increased risk of a heart attack is a ripple moving through the water — evidence of an energetic disturbance. And yet, doctors can't measure stress. Stress is an energetic phenomenon that has physical effects. Because doctors can't measure stress, they don't treat it. Medical dogma assumes the things that can be measured, such as cholesterol, are more important than those that can't, such as stress.

This focus on measuring things to diagnose disease is not specific to heart disease. In depression, medical treatment in the form of drugs is based on the idea of treating a thing (low serotonin levels). Cancer treatments are based on killing a thing, cancer cells, with toxic drugs or radiation or cutting the cancer out via surgery. Yet, health is not created by treating things. In fact, sometimes by focusing on doing something (like surgery) we ignore treatments that utilize the quantum principle (the power of no-thing), like the placebo effect.

The Baylor School of Medicine published a study in 2002 evaluating the effectiveness of different types of surgery for the treatment of knee pain. The lead author of the study, Dr. Bruce J. Moseley, a clinical associate professor of orthopedics at Baylor at the time and now Program Director, Sports Medicine Fellowship, wanted to know which type of surgery was most effective for degeneration arthritis of the knee. There are two main surgeries for this type of arthritis. In the first type, doctors shave off damaged cartilage in the knee — removing the thing thought to be irritating the joint. In the second, surgeons flush out the knee joint, once again to remove the thing causing the inflammation. Dr. Moseley wanted to know which type of surgery, shaving or flushing, was most effective in treating knee pain.

To study the effectiveness of each type of surgery, Dr. Moseley also needed what is called a control group. The control group is a group of patients who don't get either type of the intervention. In this case, the control group would get a "fake" surgery meaning they would be sedated, surgeons would make standard incisions around the joint while they act and talk as if they were conducting a real surgery. Yet, in the control group, there would no flushing of the knee or shaving of cartilage. Instead, after 40 minutes, the surgeons would then close the incisions, even though they had not done anything inside the joint — no shaving or flushing. The surgeons didn't know which type of surgery (shaving, flushing, or the placebo surgery) they would be performing until the first incision. So even with the control group, the doctors and teams prepped as if they were doing the real thing. Once scrubbed in, the surgeons got an envelope from researchers indicating which type of surgery they were to perform. The patients in the study would never know which group they were in (shaving, flushing, or placebo). Post-op, all three groups were prescribed the same recovery plan and the same rehabilitation exercises.

It turns out, the improvement in patients who got the knee shaved and flushed was about equal. What surprised Dr. Moseley, and many others, was that the patients who received the fake surgery got better as well, improving just as much as those who got the real surgery! Dr. Moseley had a sobering realization: "My skill as a surgeon had no benefit on these patients. The entire benefit of surgery for degenerative arthritis of the knee was the placebo effect."

Dr. Mosely is a nationally recognized orthopedic surgeon and expert in cartilage restoration. He was a team physician for the Houston NBA and WNBA teams and served as the team physician for the US Men's and Women's Olympic Basketball Teams.

How can this be, that the skill of a nationally recognized surgeon was useless in helping patients heal? The patients in the study all had significant arthritis. The degeneration was visible on X-ray. The patients were in pain and this pain limited their activities of daily living. They limped, they had difficulty bending their leg, they struggled to get into and out of chairs. Their arthritis was a very real disease. And yet, the placebo effect, defined as the beneficial effect produced by a drug or treatment that cannot be attributed to the procedure, was equally as effective as the actual knee surgery. That is, in all three groups the improvement of pain, range of motion, and function were the same.

How can researchers explain this fact, that those who believed they were getting real knee surgery, but in fact did not, improved just as much as groups who got the real surgery?

To answer this question, we have to understand the power of the placebo.

Placebos have been studied more than any other intervention in medicine. More than any drug, any surgery, or any medical device. Just like we saw with knee surgery, researchers evaluating the effectiveness of a drug measure the drug against a placebo. Drugs that work better than a placebo are approved and those that don't are rejected. Drugs are compared to a placebo specifically to mitigate the placebo effect we saw above. By comparing drugs to a placebo, medicine can limit non-tangible influences such as patients' beliefs and hopes from the drug, the thing, being studied.

To a drug company, the effectiveness of a placebo is a problem. To get a drug approved, you must prove the new drug works better than a placebo. The more effective the placebo, the higher the bar the drug or intervention must clear. Therefore, in medicine, patients who get better without a drug or a real surgery are a problem.

But, don't you think, if 35-75% of all patients get better from an intervention that costs virtually nothing and has no side effects, that may not be *all* bad? We are in the middle of a healthcare crisis of rising costs and declining care, patients getting sicker and sicker, rising rates of bankruptcy due to medical costs and yet we are writing off the most studied intervention ever that costs virtually nothing and has no side effects.

Is this not insane? (A word which, incidentally enough, comes from Latin roots meaning not healthy.) From a holistic viewpoint, rather than trying to eliminate the placebo effect, what if we instead tried to understand it? What if instead we were curious about it and asked, why does the placebo work?

If we did, we would find the placebo works because of holism — evidencing the Yellowstone Principle from the second chapter. In this chapter, we can add another layer to the story. There is more to creating a healthy knee than flushing or shaving the joint. Equally as powerful, as the study showed, is the patient's belief in their own healing. The power of nothing is as powerful as surgery. Yet we live in a medical idea of health that prescribes surgery as standard of care for arthritis of the knee and ignores the equally effective, safer, and less costly placebo. While factors such as rest, attention, and the benefits of physical therapy might have helped healing in those who got the placebo surgery, researchers attributed the largest portion of the patients' improvement to the placebo effect. This is not to say that fake, placebo knee surgery should be the new standard of care of arthritis of the knee. But also — this is not to say that it should *not* be the new standard of care. If there is another intervention that costs less, has fewer side effects, and results in equal improvement for the patient, wouldn't that intervention merit a closer look?

Just because the placebo effect doesn't fit into the dogma of disease care is not reason enough to dismiss it out of hand. Following the medical idea of health, we make the mistake that all that matters is matter, ignoring the less tangible aspects of health including beliefs, emotions, and hope. And that is the lesson of this story, that faith and hope are as powerful a force for healing as surgery.

The power of the placebo is not limited to sham knee surgeries as above. If you give a patient a placebo, a sugar pill, at least 30% of patients get better. The United States Department of Health and Human Services in 1999 studied the power of the placebo in depression. It found that half of severely depressed patients improved taking drugs, while 32% improved with the placebo. Three years later, Professor Irving Kirsh at the University of Connecticut published research that found up to 80% of the effect of antidepressants, as measured in clinical trials, could be attributed to the placebo effect. But the placebo effect does not just help depression, or conditions that are "in our head." In fact, the placebo effect has been shown to be helpful in almost every type of disease.

According to popular thinking, depression is caused by a chemical imbalance in the brain. This theory, however, like the theory of the atom, has never been proven. No one has ever measured the chemicals inside someone's brain to diagnose them with depression. Instead, brain chemicals become a convenient explanation as medicine looks to implicate a tangible thing in the pathology of depression. Yet the placebo effect might explain 80%of the effect of antidepressants. Which leads to the question, what is more powerful, matter or energy?

In fact, the reason we know little about the causes of depression is because we are looking for a physical, tangible cause. We are looking at the chemicals of the brain to tell the story of depression yet, the chemicals of the brain are not the cause of depression. Even if they do change as scientists theorize, they may only be the result. Changes in serotonin levels may only be ripples in the water. The question that begs to be asked is, why is serotonin low in the first place? And is this a serotonin issue in and of itself or an adaption by the body to its environment? Is it a ripple we observe because a pebble has fallen?

While depression has many causes, a major contributor to depression is loss — loss of loved ones, loss of job, loss of love, loss of purpose. Loss is a very real thing, although it can't be touched. Despite the fact we can't touch loss, it has a very tangible effect on the brain and body. It creates ripples in the body that manifest as disease. We understand loss can cause depression, but we still treat depression as a deficiency of a thing, serotonin, with a tangible treatment, that of a prescription medication.

While this is not to say that things don't matter, what is missing from the medical idea of health is the power of the intangible to cause disease. Because you would treat depression very differently if you thought it was caused by a chemical imbalance (that could supposedly be treated with a drug), than by an unexpected or traumatic life event someone was trying to cope with.

Research has shown that exercise is as effective at treating depression as taking two antidepressant medications. A placebo is 80% as effective as most drugs. And yet, when it comes to treating depression, medicine ignores proven, free therapies, like placebos and exercise and counseling to manage loss, and instead prescribes drugs as standard of care. If your goal is to create health, hope and exercise and the healthy processing of life are of great benefit to any patient — depressed or otherwise. If your goal is to treat disease following the medical approach, you would prescribe a drug and see the patient at their next visit.

Why would medical idea of disease not utilize an intervention that helps a third of all patients and costs nothing? If a doctor had told me when I was seven years old that a near-free therapy without side effects that had a 30-80% chance of helping my headaches was available, I would have signed up for it in a second. Especially when my other options were brain surgery or prescription drugs that were not helping me.

It is hard, if not impossible, to embrace the placebo effect within the medical idea of health where no-thing equals nothing. Yet, the effectiveness of the placebo evidences its power. The placebo effect is a reminder of the power of the intangible to create health.

The quantum principle is not totally foreign to medical care. Traditional medicine does incorporate the quantum principle in limited aspects. One example is an electrocardiogram, EKG. This is a medical test of the heart that measures its electrical activity. Said another way, the EKG measures the flow of energy through the heart. Similarly, an EEG, an electroencephalogram, is a medical test that measures the energy of the brain. In fact, even X-rays, CT scans, and MRIs all measure subtle differences in energy in the body. They don't measure something tangible, instead they measure no-thing (energy). The medical system also uses the quantum principle to treat disease. One such example is lithotripsy, a treatment for kidney stones which uses ultrasound waves to break apart the stone while still in the kidney making it easier for the patient to pass. Each of these use the principle of energy to diagnose or treat disease.

This is just the beginning of what is possible.

If we are not made of things and are in fact made of energy, wouldn't it make sense that the energetic domain is the most powerful healing domain?

Atoms are made of energy. The subatomic particles are expressions of energy. Our nervous system runs off energy. Because of this, mastering the energetic domain is the next frontier in health.

Oxford biophysicist C. W. F. McClare, as quoted in the *Biology of Belief,* concludes that energetic stimuli in biological systems, such as electromagnetic frequencies, are 100 times more efficient in relaying environmental information than physical signals such as hormones, neurotransmitters, and growth factors. With this he says that our body is 100 times more receptive to energy than it is to things. Since most medical treatments are pharmaceuticals and thus based on physical signals, his conclusion opens up amazing possibilities of therapies and treatments 100 times more powerful than what we now know.

It is a testament to the fact that no-thing is more powerful than just about everything.

Mark Twain was not a doctor, but he might as well have been one when he wrote, "It happened slowly, then all of the sudden." He was writing about the process of going bankrupt, but that process extends far beyond personal finances. In fact, long before we see the ripples of disease, the heart attack, the cancer, the headache, a stone first fell in the water disrupting balance. Without finding the initial cause, we are doomed to forever treat ripples.

In the medical system, if there is no-thing to treat, the doctors are often out of options. Dr. Wolfe sent me back to my pediatrician with a recommendation to continue imaging the cyst to make sure the thing was not a problem. I had another dozen or so MRIs over the next 10 years. Each new set of images was compared to the earlier studies looking for a change. As long as it didn't grow, the risks of surgery would not be worth the reward. But what could I do in the meantime? Without a thing to treat, my doctors didn't have a clear treatment plan for me. Even though my symptoms varied greatly over the 10 years, the mass in my head, the suspected cause, never changed. As a result, my doctors decided the mass was not the cause of my headaches. As a patient, where did this leave me? In a place where I had more questions than answers. In a place with a condition that medicine could not find a cause. In a place where I faced the reality that my headaches were caused either by something that had not been found or by something that was not actually a thing.

The intangible is a surprisingly strong force to create health or disease. Its power extends beyond knee pain and depression and headaches to touch even one of the most common conditions in the world — obesity.

We all know the cause of obesity, right? Too much food and not enough exercise.

But what if the obesity epidemic is not caused by too much food and too little exercise? This is the story of one man who dared to ask this question, and the principles of health he discovered in the process.

Vincent Felitti led Kaiser Permanente's Department of Preventative Medicine in San Diego in the 1980s. Part of his job was to oversee their obesity clinic in San Diego, California. People as little as 30 pounds overweight could visit the clinic, but the clinic was intended for those who were 100-600 pounds overweight. Felitti was troubled that the clinic had a dropout rate of 50%. He wanted to understand why the patients were leaving the program. Through interviews with dropouts, he found that all those who left the program were successfully losing weight. Why, Felitti then wondered, were patients dropping out of the program if they were losing weight? As he probed deeper, he discovered that the majority of the 286 dropouts he interviewed experienced childhood sexual abuse. They told Feliti they were not obese because they didn't know what to eat or the importance of exercise. Instead, they told Felitti, they were using food to handle the pain of abuse.

As he reviewed the health history of the clinic's patients Felitti was shocked. "I had assumed that people who were 400, 500, 600 pounds overweight would be getting heavier and heavier year after year." Felitti says, "In 2,000 people, I didn't see it once." When the patients gained weight, they gained it abruptly and then their weight stabilized. If they lost weight, they often regained all of it, or more, over a short time.

Being overweight, Felitti found, was not the problem. It was actually the *solution* to an even bigger problem. Like others use alcohol or drugs, Felitti found his obese patients used food to feel better and soothe their emotions (anxiety, fear, and pain). Often, the patients craved foods highest in refined carbohydrates, processed sugars, and fats. They used food to solve the very real yet intangible stress, fear, and anxiety they felt. After the 286 initial interviews in which many patients described the connection between abuse and obesity, Felitti was intrigued, but not yet convinced. He wanted more proof.

His curiosity eventually grew into the Adverse Childhood Experiences (ACE) Study. Felitti partnered with Robert Anda of the Centers of Disease Control and Prevention (CDC). The two would go on to interview 17,337 members of Kaiser Permanente, a Health Maintenance Organization (HMO), expanding on the initial reports of sexual abuse to investigate the presence of 10 types of childhood trauma in obese patients. The 10 types of childhood trauma were:

1. Physical Abuse
2. Sexual Abuse
3. Emotional Abuse
4. Physical Neglect
5. Emotional Neglect
6. Exposure to Domestic Violence
7. Household Substance Abuse
8. Household Mental Illness
9. Parental Separation or Divorce

10. Incarcerated Household Member

For each adverse experience in a person's childhood, they scored a point. Just as Felitti found in his initial interviews, a definite connection existed between adverse childhood experiences (ACE) and obesity. Further, the correlation was linear, meaning the higher the patient's ACE score, the more likely the patient was to be obese. The research correlated to Felitti's initial findings and interviews: obesity and overeating were not the problem; they were the solution. The problem was the emotional scars of what he termed adverse childhood experiences. The patients were using food to handle the pain.

And yet, this is just the beginning of the story. The real bombshell was uncovering that the ACE score (how many of the 10 types of childhood trauma they experienced) also correlated with many common diseases including heart disease, cancer, chronic lung disease, depression, substance abuse, suicide, and a shortened lifespan. For example, compared with an ACE score of zero, an ACE score of four was associated with a 700% increase in alcoholism, a 200% increase in cancer, and a 400% increase in emphysema. An ACE score above six was associated with a 3,000% increase in attempted suicide. Further, as the number of ACEs someone experiences increase, so does their risk of fetal death, illicit drug use, liver disease, risk for intimate partner violence, sexually transmitted diseases, smoking, and unintended pregnancy.

Perhaps, every doctor who has patients dealing with obesity, cancer, heart disease, suicide, emphysema, alcoholism, substance abuse, infection, and mental health really needs to be treating emotional health. All of these diseases are correlated with non-physical causes.

According to the World Health Organization, the study's findings within the United States reflect a truth around the world. Research confirming these findings has been done on patient populations on five continents.

Through his research, Felitti discovered a principle of health hiding in plain sight. What he uncovered is a smoking gun in our current health epidemic. A strong, dose dependent correlation between the most stressful events of childhood and health and disease risk through the rest of life. What he stumbled on, of course, was the quantum principle.

The power of this research is that there is now a new and exciting avenue to pursue in the treatment of obesity and creation of health. One especially empowering considering current treatments are failing. Obesity is now considered a global epidemic. One which threatens to leave today's children as the first generation to have a shorter lifespan than their parents.

Felitti's findings and the quantum principle help explain why the disease care system worldwide struggles with obesity. The struggle emanates from only looking at things as the cause of obesity and ignoring the power of emotional health. The medical system attempts to treat obesity by treating its effects and ignoring the underlying cause — the unhandled trauma of adverse experiences that drives patients to soothe their pain with toxic foods. The quantum principle tells us we need to heed the words of McClare that no-thing is more powerful than a thing.

I do feel obliged to add here that we need not absolve the fast-food (fast poison) companies, soft drink or processed food manufacturers selling toxic, sweetened trans-fat food stuffs. This has no place in creating a healthy body. But what if we accept the quantum principle as true and look one level deeper at the problem? What does a body under stress crave? It craves energy to survive the stressor. A body stuck in a stress response craves energy dense, high calorie foods. Which foods are quickest to provide in calories? Refined carbohydrates: Sugar, bread, pasta, donuts, cookies, candy, and soft drinks. Which foods provide the most calories? Those highest in fats. While not all fats are bad, and in fact healthy fats are a vital part of health, when we are stressed, we don't often crave fresh salmon or olives. Instead, we reach for the worst kinds of fats, those that are heavily processed and refined such as in processed junk food. Add to this a craving for caffeine to boost energy levels and you have the recipe for most of what is wrong with the Standard American Diet. Too many processed carbohydrates, too many junk fats, and too much caffeine artificially stimulating the body. We as a world are eating like people stuck in the middle of a painful stress response. And, according to Felitti, this is because many of us are.

In the short term, the stress response is an appropriate response. Eating carbohydrates or fats before running for your life is not a bad trade off. They may very well give you a short-term energy boost. The problem comes when we are under such stress that we are eating the equivalent of a half a candy bar (or soda, or refined carbohydrate creation or sugary-sweet beverage) every few hours for months upon years upon decades. All without burning the extra energy we crave to solve the stress. A healthy stress response is short lived, present at the moment of stress which we optimally handle and then return the body to a state of ease.

Today, the fight-or-flight response is triggered, not by attacks from wild animals or moments of famine, like our ancestors faced, but by feelings of loneliness, ACEs, depression, loss, fear and anxiety among others. In the chapter titled Olympic Strength Principle, we will discuss more on the effects of stress on health and how to transform stress from a negative into a positive. Finding healthy ways to deal with stress is more important than ever before. Unlike our ancestors' problems, stressors today, often emotional, tend to last longer than a transient bear attack. The understanding that many live for decades under stress must reframe how we understand obesity and food cravings specifically, and health generally.

The effects of stress are covered more deeply in the next chapter. For now, stress is but one example of a non-physical cause that has very physical effects. Yet, despite this very real connection, it is a connection that our medical disease care system largely ignores.

I had recently read about the ACE study and Felitti's work when Sam entered the office. As she sat down on the table, she wanted to lose weight.

Weighing 342 pounds at a height of 5'2", she knew she was very overweight, and she had struggled for years to get her body to look the way she wanted. She had tried many times to lose weight. Sometimes she would lose weight only to later gain it back. Often, she would gain back even more than she lost. On the first visit, Sam also shared her other health concerns including an irregular menstrual cycle, back pain, swelling in her feet, and low energy levels. But she told me, her priority was to get her weight under control. At age 45, she was ready to make a change.

She wanted to lose weight — a lot of weight. The look in her eye said she was embarrassed — even scared — to honestly share how much weight she wanted to lose. At first, she said she would love to lose 50 pounds. Her "dream," she later told me, would be to lose 100 pounds. Almost a year later she confessed her true goal was to lose 142 pounds and break under 200 pounds for the first time in decades.

As we discussed her health history, I was curious about her pattern of weight gain, wondering if it was a long gradual gain or a period of quick jumps as Felitti described. It was not gradual, but instead a few jumps of 30-60 pounds that got her to where she was today.

We discussed her most recent jump in weight three years ago. I asked what had been going on in her life prior to that most recent jump. As I did, I looked into her eyes and she stared back into mine. Terror crossed her now pale face. She couldn't speak. I waited. Soon, tears started to roll down her face. "Give me the tissues," she said. As she wiped the tears from her eyes, she told the story of being forcibly raped and beaten by a former partner. During the rape, her former partner pulled a gun on her threatening her life and the lives of her children if she didn't do what he said. She was overwhelmed with emotion and pain. I asked her if there was a moment of shock connected to the rape? When she answered yes, I then asked her a series of questions to help her process the shock, similar to the process I ran with Lisa, whose psoriasis flared up after her boyfriend's infidelity. As part of the process, I asked her to describe the incident, including the moods and emotions frozen in the shock. "This shit is hard for me to talk about," she told me that day, but she bravely decided to press on describing the incident, with the aid of a few tissues and an occasional joke. We especially focused on the locked-up moods in the shock, which were anger and rage. Within a few days of running the shock, she lost nine pounds. The emotional pain that was weighing on her, once released, led to quick release in physical weight as well. Two weeks later, we processed another shock that preceded an earlier jump in weight, and she lost another eight pounds in the following two weeks. Combined, after processing two shocks, she dropped 17 pounds in less than a month.

Over the next 18 months, we combined exercise (which started with walking 4-5 minutes per day) and dietary changes with processing other shocks from her life. Where this differs from the findings of Felitti is that the shocks Sam identified were not shocks from her childhood, but they certainly were adverse experiences.

While Felitti's research didn't extend to adverse adult experiences, in my experience the mechanics of shock and stress function the same way, no matter the age they occur. A painful incident that causes fears, anxieties, and hurt is awful at any age. The first lesson of Felitti's work, and Sam's story as well, is the power of emotional shocks to affect our physical health. This is the bad news. The second lesson — the good news — is that these scars are reversable. While we can't change the past, we can absolutely change how the past affects us in the present.

As we process the moods or emotions that are stuck in the shock, we can reverse the emotional scars and halt the increased risk of disease. As Sam did this, her health continued to improve. As I write this, she is down about 70 pounds over 16 months, in line with a very healthy weight loss pattern of a pound per week. More importantly, the physical weight loss is a reflection of her improved emotional health. By addressing the intangible, we can improve the tangible markers of health in a very real way.

When I think back to the fifth-grade classroom, how I wish I had known what I know now. Sure, a basic understanding of quantum physics is a tad ambitious for a fifth grader. But, imagine if I had understood that the atom is 99.996% empty space, I could have confidently walked into the class and turned in a project of nothing. A model of nothing, with no-things making it up, would have been an infinitely more correct model of the atom. When Mrs. Stanczyk asked me why I didn't do the project, I could have confidently looked her in the eyes and said, "I did do my homework. It's right here" (gesturing toward empty space). "Don't you see?" I would have said. "The best model of the atom is actually nothing. It's all energy."

What I wouldn't learn for another two decades is how the lessons from the atom would profoundly affect my health. I spent far too long in a medical idea of health looking for things that were causing my headaches, without understanding that we live in a world built from energy, not things.

Ultimately, there was never a "thing" that a doctor could point to as a cause for my headaches. What I didn't realize until later was how many other patients are like me. How many other patients walk into their doctor's office with a pain, or irregular bowels, or fatigue, or any other symptom only for the doctor to tell them, "Your blood work looks fine" or "You look healthy to me" or "I am not sure what is going on with you"? Sometimes the doctor's response is a prescription for an antidepressant, implying the disease is all in the patient's head. In cases like this, the doctor is close; their instinct that a physical symptom has an emotional cause is one worth exploring. However, the solution I would propose would embrace the quantum principle, helping the client to process through the stressor rather than numbing it with a drug.

This chapter's lesson is that we live in a quantum world, and because we do, we can't limit medical care to always looking for things. The water ripples because of energy, not the other way around.

Einstein once said that the field is the sole governing agent of the particle. With this he was saying that energetic fields control particles or, said another way, energy controls things. When ripples move through a pond, it is the waves of energy that move the water. Felitti's research tells us that the energetic stress of ACEs are the field which affect the health of the particle, the body. In Sam's case, by processing the energetic shock and releasing the anger and fear trapped in the incident, positive changes rippled through her body. This same principle applies to all disease, and all aspects of health. We live in a quantum universe and by accepting this fact, we can move from treating the ripples to calming the energetic waves — creating health at its source.

Which takes me back to my story...

*While I didn't understand how it all worked, I knew I was getting better. In the two years since my first appointment in Atlanta, I had continued chiropractic care and supplements to help with the headaches. While many in my life told me I was crazy for trying something different, I felt I had no choice. It was worth it, but it was not easy. My health regimen included taking handfuls of supplements each day, going regularly for chiropractic care, and being fastidious with my diet. I strictly avoided all foods with refined and processed sugars in them (which happens to be a lot of them) and most dairy. Because of this, I never went out to eat by choice. It was just too hard. If I went out to eat because of obligation, like a family celebration, I would always custom order a meal and ask many questions about the ingredients and how it was prepared. I was so sensitive that if the waiter or kitchen messed up, and some sugar or dairy or some other problematic ingredient ended up in the meal, I might be knocked out with a headache for days. Eating out simply wasn't worth the risk. I avoided it as much as I could.*

*Because of this, I learned how to cook. Nothing fancy, but it was worth it to me to be 100% sure of everything I put into my body. If I went over to friends' houses or away to travel, I preferred to bring my own food than chance it.*

*Through it all, I knew I was getting better. This is what made all the extra effort worth it to me, now a sophomore in high school. About two years and six or seven trips to see the holistic doctor in Atlanta later, my headaches were so much better. They were not gone but compared to the pain and agony I had experienced for years, my on-*

*going recovery felt like a miracle.*

*I was able to play sports in high school. Plans with friends were not made with a constant proviso of "if I feel up to it". By my estimates, my headaches were at least 80% better. For me this felt miraculous.*

*Unfortunately, the story doesn't end here.*

*Because I was so much better, I fell into my old patterns of thinking from the medical idea of health. That is, if you are not sick, you don't need to go see a doctor. Because of this, (I mean, I was better, right?), I stopped going to see the holistic doctor. I would still take some supplements and still maintained a good diet. I thought that would be enough. I was wrong.*

*Not only did the headaches come back, by my junior year of high school, they came back with a vengeance. In fact, the headache I wrote about at the beginning, the three-day headache that trapped me in my bed, happened only after I was better and then crashed. This incredible improvement in my headaches and then subsequent worsening crushed me. The headaches were now more painful and more frequent than they had ever been. How could I be so stupid? I wondered. Had I wasted all that time and progress? I felt horrible, worse than ever. The pain of the headaches was only made worse by the knowledge that just a few months earlier I had felt great. Seeing the light of two years of health only made the darkness of the headaches' return so much more crushing.*

*With the benefit of hindsight, I can see that this crash*

*taught me three valuable lessons. The first was the supplements and health are not like drugs and medicine.*

*You see, raised in the medical idea of disease, I was used to taking drugs when I was sick, and then not needing them when I was healthy. When I applied this same idea, to only take care of myself when I am sick and not when I am healthy, it produced disastrous results. I learned that just as I could create health by a series of correct steps and actions, by abandoning those steps and actions I was also abandoning my journey toward health. To sum up this first lesson, treating disease might be episodic — take a drug and see a doctor when you are sick — the creation of health is a constant journey.*

*The second lesson I learned is one of empathy. Because of this experience, I would develop a deep empathy for patients who had the similar experience of a series of wins and improvements only to later crash down. After glimpsing the joy of health, the return of disease and symptoms often leaves patients feeling worse than before. I get it.*

*I also learned a third lesson. Once you have walked the road to health once, even if you get knocked backward and feel worse again, it is almost always easier to climb the second time, because you already know the path, the pitfalls, and prize at the end.*

"The greatest mistake in the treatment of diseases is that there are physicians for the body, and physicians for the soul, although the two cannot be separated."

**PLATO (428-348 BC)**

---

# CHAPTER 5
# OLYMPIC STRENGTH PRINCIPLE

## How Titanic Problems Lead
## to Olympic Strength

The question of what brought down the Titanic, in the months after the disaster, captured the attention of the world. What sunk the unsinkable? In the end, official blame was placed on the deceased Captain Smith. The ship was going too fast considering the icy conditions. Because of this, it did not have time to avoid the iceberg. Upon impact, the iceberg ripped a hole in the hull and the mighty ship went down, in one piece, to the bottom of the Atlantic.

That was the official story for over 70 years until Robert Ballard, who dreamed of finding the wreckage of the *Titanic* for as long as he could remember, found the ship in 1986. When the *Titanic* was located, the bow and stern of the ship were discovered over a mile and a half apart

— contradicting the official narrative that the *Titanic* went down in one piece. This new evidence indicated that the bow of the ship, weighed down by the water rushing into her six watertight compartments, leaned forward and to the right. This eventually tilted the stern 45 degrees into the air, lifting its three giant propellers out of the water until the hull, overwhelmed by the strain, snapped in two.

This new theory of how the *Titanic* sank centers on stress. In science, stress is defined as pressure or tension exerted on a material object. Over the last three and a half decades, material scientists have searched the wreckage for signs of physical stress that caused the disaster. In short, under the stress of striking an iceberg, how did the ship fail?

At first, researchers questioned the integrity of the steel hull. To test this theory, material scientists tested a cigarette-sized piece of steel, recovered from the *Titanic*'s hull at the bottom of the Atlantic. Would the steel of the *Titanic* bend and flex under pressure, like high-quality steel should, or would it snap in two? Under the stress of testing, modern high-quality steel flexed and bent into a V shape. It did not break. The steel recovered from the wreckage of the *Titanic* snapped in two. Brittle steel is the difference between an iceberg denting the hull by deforming its shape and the iceberg ripping the hull open. This difference was attributed to the difference in the chemical makeup of the two pieces of steel. The *Titanic*'s steel was found to have high levels of oxygen and sulfur, both of which weaken the steel and create a more brittle hull.

Yet, it is not just a high oxygen and high sulfur content that cause steel to fail instead of flex under stress. Two other factors, low temperatures and a high impact collision, also contributed to the failure of *Titanic*'s hull. On the night of April 14ᵗʰ, all four stressors were present: high oxygen content in the hull, high sulfur content in the hull, near freezing waters, and a high impact collision with an iceberg. It is noteworthy that all four had to be present to cause failure. Without the high impact, the low temperatures and weakened steel were not enough to cause problems, as evidenced by the *Titanic's* safe journey pre-iceberg.

Metallurgists Tim Foecke and Jennifer Hooper McCarthy investigated the rivets that held the ship's steel hull together as a possible point of failure. Specifically, they found poorer quality rivets in the part of the hull where the *Titanic* struck an iceberg. Weaker rivets, made of iron, were used in the bow and stern of the ship while stronger steel rivets were used in the center. In addition, they found higher concentrations of "slag," a residue of smelting that weakens iron, in those rivets. The parts of the *Titanic* with the stronger steel rivets survived the collision while, upon impact, the weaker iron rivets in the bow popped. This then ripped open the hull and sped up the sinking of the *Titanic*. Interestingly, the flooding stopped at the point in the hull where the steel rivets began.

Ultimately, material scientists say, the sinking of the *Titanic* can be understood as a weakened structure overwhelmed by stress.

In bodies, like ships, a weakened structure overwhelmed by stress explains much of our current disaster. As mentioned earlier, medical textbooks say 60-80% of all disease is caused by stress. The Centers for Disease Control and Prevention says 75% of all doctors' visits are for conditions caused by stress.

It is when we hit the icebergs of our lives, faced with extreme stress, that our weaknesses come to view. Sitting in the harbor, the *Titanic's* iron rivets, high in slag, and weakened steel did not fail. However, they were potential problems silently lurking, not yet given voice by the presence of stress. It is the same with our body. Sailing through life, in periods of low stress, the potential weaknesses of our body are not yet evident. Even if we appear to be symptom free in the calm waters of life, we cannot mistakenly confuse this with health. Only when we encounter the major stressors of life do we get a fuller picture of the integrity and health of the body.

In medicine, the absence of disease is often mistaken for health. This is a fallacy. The *Titanic* on April 10th was symptom free, but it had major problems that, quite literally, lingered both above and below the surface. We must not confuse the absence of symptoms as health. Without adequate nutrients needed to heal and repair, we cannot survive the inevitable stressors of life. Yet, on the contrary, with adequate nutrition, we can strengthen our body not only to handle these inevitable stressors, but also to grow stronger because of them. Said another way, the slag rivets were a problem the whole time. They were always weakening the structure of the *Titanic*. But, although they were a potential problem, there were not yet a disaster.

On September 20, 1911, two and a half years before the *Titanic* met her fate, another ship, the *Olympic*, was leaving the same South Hampton port on her way to New York. Like the *Titanic*, when this ship hit the water, it was the largest manmade moving object in the world. As the ship left the harbor and turned toward New York, it passed a second ship, a British war ship, the HMS *Hawke*. As the largest ship in the world turned, the much smaller *Hawke* was unintentionally drawn toward the larger ship, as if by suction, by the larger ship's giant propellers. This caused the bow of the *Hawke* to collide with the much larger ship tearing two large holes in the *Olympic*'s hull, one above and one below the water line.

The trip to New York was canceled. The vessel faced two months of repairs. These repairs ultimately made the *Olympic* stronger than it was before. Thankfully, no lives were lost as a result of the incident.

While all collisions — whether with another ship, an iceberg, or something else — result in pressure or tension exerted on a material object, this ship, the *Olympic* went on to sail for another 24 years. The structure of the *Titanic*, of course, was overwhelmed by its first collision. The lesson of the *Olympic* is that stress does not have to be a bad thing. In fact, stress can be a catalyst to help us grow stronger. Stress does not have to sink us; it can make us stronger. This is Olympic Strength.

In the body, stress comes in many forms. Exercise causes the release of stress hormones, the tearing down of muscle and physical exhaustion. Infection can lead to injury, disease, and death. Emotional loss can lead to sadness, tears, and depression. All stressors have the potential to sink us. Yet, they also have the potential to make us stronger. Exercise after tearing down muscles triggers the body to build the muscles back stronger. Exercise also strengthens bones and results in a more resilient cardiovascular system. Infection leads to the development of natural immunity and a more resilient immune system. The stress of a loss can strengthen our own coping skills and better help us help others going through the same grief.

The question for each of us is, how can we use the stresses in our lives to get stronger, like the *Olympic*, and not sink, like the *Titanic*? In short, in response to stress, how can we develop *Olympic* strength and not become a *Titanic* disaster?

As we saw last chapter, traditional medicine and the medical idea of health practically ignore the intangible (believing everything that matters is matter). To create health, we must embrace the quantum principle. Stress is the most powerful factor, tangible or intangible, affecting our health. Yet, in practice it remains hidden in plain sight. As we saw with the research on Adverse Childhood Experiences, medicine treats people for heart disease, obesity, and cancer yet ignores the stressors that underlies all three. With this, the medical idea of health makes the same mistake as Captain Smith and the crew of the *Titanic*, allowing false perceptions to cloud their judgement. As with the *Titanic*, this misperception threatens disaster, if it has not already struck.

The word stress is often used and poorly defined. In fact, in my years of schooling and reading medical books, I have not found a medical definition that really explains what stress is. A typical medical dictionary might define stress as a physiological disturbance or damage caused by adverse circumstances. This definition has many words, but it doesn't say much. That is why earlier I referenced the physics definition of stress — pressure or tension exerted on a material object. It strikes me as a more practical definition.

A second description of stress that I find helpful comes from the 10th anniversary edition of *Eat, Pray, Love*. In the Prologue, Elizabeth Gilbert writes:

"The word stress comes from the Latin word for compression, and that compression is what prematurely ages us — compacting us, physically and emotionally, into a feeling of frailty and brokenness."

A key part of this definition is the idea of stress affecting the body in a physical way. What then, I wondered, is the force that compresses us?

The answer, I believe, is the must-not-be experienced moods or emotions in our lives. The resistance to these moods creates energetic ripples that manifest in disease. While the exact resisted moods are unique for each of us, examples may include the overwhelm we feel at the office, the anxiety we feel when separated from a partner, and the uncertainty in the face of a challenge. In fact, there could be thousands of situations that trigger stress. But what actually triggers the stress is not the experience in and of itself, but instead our resistance to experiencing the moods it contains.

In reaction to an unwanted mood — let's say the loss of a loved one — we might feel guilt or remorse or sadness. We often try to ignore these moods, to bury them, stuff them down, or pretend they don't exist. We might try not to think about the loss. Yet each of these decisions, to ignore or bury or pretend or not think, creates energetic waves. Each choice causes ripples in the body.

Until we are present with the loss, filling the pain with love, those waves of energy are still there, even if we are not thinking of them. We know this is true because if someone says just the right phrase to us, if we pass by a certain street or restaurant, or we sit in stillness with our own thoughts, the rush of emotion comes back. We cry, we swear, our heart rate rises, our mind races, we can't sleep. The emotion that we thought was long gone in the past arrives very much in the present. Our past stresses and anxieties become our present illnesses.

In the emotional world, what we resist, persists. These resisted moods and emotions trigger a stress response that is intended to be short term (think running away from a bear). Yet, if the source of stress is not handled, the stress response persists. An unhandled short-term stressor becomes a long-term problem. This is another lesson of the Adverse Childhood Experiences study. Past stress creates present disease. What holds the trauma in place, whether that trauma be an ACE or something else, is the unhandled moods in the incident. These must-not-be-experienced items act like glue that holds the stressor in place, allowing the past upsets and future anxieties to trigger disease in the present.

To transform the stressor from a catalyst of disease to a catalyst for Olympic strength, we must work through the must-not-be-experienced moods that create the pressure. We must be present with them, with a willingness to both experience and create these moods. As we do this, the must-not-be-experienced moods which cement the compression in place release. With this, we can then return to the present moment, releasing the stress of the past.

While in the world of the *Titanic*, the stressors are physical in nature — like an iceberg in the Atlantic ripping open the hull — in bodies, the stressors are often intangible. They include the heaviness of loss, the strain of long hours, the weight of expectations and the pressure of an approaching deadline. Isn't it interesting that many of the words we use for stress (*heaviness, strain, weight, pressure)* come from the vocabulary of physics?

If the Centers for Disease Control and Prevention is correct, and stress causes 60 to 80% of all disease, it raises the question, how? In science the first step to determine causation is to first determine correlation. To explain the difference, think of wet sidewalks and people with umbrellas. Research would show that those two factors are correlated, meaning the more people carry umbrellas, the more likely the sidewalks are to be wet. Yet, it would also show that wetter the sidewalks are, the more likely there are to be people carrying umbrellas. This is correlation. It shows a connection between two variables. Felitti's research establishes a correlation between ACE and disease.

The next step, establishing causation, is harder. In our example above, we know that carrying umbrellas doesn't cause wet sidewalks, just as wet sidewalks don't cause people to carry umbrellas. Instead, both factors are caused by a third factor: rain. In this way, researchers remind us, we must be careful not to confuse correlation and causation. Just because two things occur together, like wet sidewalks and umbrellas, doesn't mean that one caused the other. Both could be caused by a third factor, in this case, rain.

When it comes to stress, many studies, like Felitti's, establish a correlation between stress and disease. To establish cause is something different entirely. One principle that researchers use to establish causation is to look for a plausible mechanism that would explain how one variable causes the other. We reject people carrying umbrellas as the cause of wet sidewalks because there is no known mechanism for why an umbrella would cause a wet sidewalk. Unless these umbrellas were equipped with a sprinkler system, there is no reason to expect one to cause the other. In contrast, with rain, we accept that idea as there is a plausible mechanism to explain its ability to cause wet sidewalks.

With stress then, we must look for a biologically plausible mechanism. How might the stress of a childhood experience, using our current understanding of biology, cause disease in the body?

To address the question of biologic plausibility, we have to introduce you to cortisol. Cortisol is a steroid hormone produced by the body in response to stress. It is studied by researchers and measured by doctors because cortisol is a tangible manifestation of intangible stress. Cortisol is produced in the body by the adrenal glands, two pea-sized organs that sit just on top of each kidney, in response to stress.

If we can draw a line between cortisol, the body's main stress hormone, and many of our most common diseases, we can establish a biologically plausible mechanism connecting the two.

In this section, we will examine how cortisol explains many of our most common diseases.

**Osteoporosis** – Cortisol levels inhibit bone formation, leading to osteoporosis. It does this in a few ways including stimulating the breakdown of bones as well as reducing the absorption of calcium from the intestines. Cortisol also slows the synthesis of collagen — one of the building blocks of bone. The end result of elevated cortisol is less bone formation.

**Digestion issues** – Cortisol helps activate the stress side of the nervous system. Once activated, the cortisol-induced stress cascade decreases blood flow to the stomach and digestive organs, resulting in decreased stomach acid. This leads to a variety of digestive issues including acid reflux, heartburn, and indigestion. Chronic stress can also lead to increased gut permeability (i.e. leaky gut) as well as inflammation of the gut. Elevated cortisol also impairs the healing and repair of the stomach lining, increasing the likelihood of stomach ulcers.

**Autoimmune Disease** – Previously, autoimmune diseases were thought to be caused by an inability of the immune system to differentiate between its own cells and invading cells. Without this ability, the immune system would then attack the body, resulting in autoimmune disease. However, new research indicates that autoimmune disease does not develop without the body simultaneously releasing danger signals in response to stress. In short, we now understand the development of autoimmune disease requires a body under stress.

**Hormonal Issues** – In response to stress, the body makes less testosterone, less estrogen, and less DHEA, the body's anti-aging hormone. Thus, we can understand stress as an important contributing factor to many hormonal disorders in women, both pre- and post-menopausal, as well as low testosterone symptoms in men.

**Obesity** – Remember the work of Felitti who found having three or more ACEs raised the risk of obesity by 400 percent? As mentioned previously, the link between obesity and ACEs can be connected by cortisol. A body under stress craves energy — the energy needed fuels the body's response to stress. Under stress, bodies crave instant energy (think sugar and fat). In addition, cortisol leads to the buildup of fat around the abdomen.

Not only does cortisol explain many of our most common diseases, but it also explains the 10 most common causes of death. While we already mentioned the medical disease care system is the number one cause of death, the CDC and medical textbooks attribute 60-80% of all doctors' visits to diseases of stress. Thus, a majority of the time stress is what gets us into the disease care system and exposes us to the risks of traditional medical care. In addition, stress and cortisol contribute to the following causes of death as well.

1. **Heart Disease** – Elevated cortisol can lead to a buildup of plaque in the arteries (atherosclerosis), especially if combined with an unhealthy diet and sedentary living. Elevated cortisol levels also promote elevated cholesterol and triglyceride levels as well as high blood pressure — all three of which increase the risk of heart attack and stroke. In fact, the day after the death of a loved one, the risk of a heart attack is 21 times higher than normal, and six times higher the week following the loss. Why? Plaque has not changed significantly in one day. Neither has cardiovascular fitness nor diet. What has changed drastically is stress. While poor lifestyle choices load the gun, stress pulls the trigger creating disease.

2. **Cancer** – Studies have found a link between elevated cortisol levels and immune system suppression (specifically suppression of natural killer (NK) cells which both prevent and destroy metastasis). Because of this, elevated cortisol is linked to tumor development. Also, chronic stress leads to chronic inflammation which further weakens the immune system. Doctors have noted a stress-cancer connection going as far back as the second century when the Greek physician Galen noted cancer was

more common in melancholy patients than cheerful ones. Mark Doolittle, PhD, of Stanford University writes that doctors in the 17th and 18th century frequently noted cancer cases were preceded by a mental depression, anxiety, deferred hope, and disappointment. More recently, Doolittle cites the work of Lawrence LeShan who studied the lives of more than 500 cancer patients and found a distinct emotional life-history pattern in 76% of cancer patients and in only 10% of the control group. A life-history pattern in which the cancer was preceded by loss and the bottling up of emotions such as anger, hurt, disappointment.

3. **Accidents / Unintentional Injuries** – Anyone who has ever been in an argument realizes that often it is only *after* the argument is over, when you calm down, that you think of your best point. (I should have said …) Ever wonder why? The reason is stress changes blood flow in the brain, away from the prefrontal cortex which regulates rational thought and toward the more primitive and reactionary parts of the brain, the brain stem and cerebellum. When this happens, we think less and react more. This results in less presence and more accidents. Research confirms this trend as when stress levels rise, so do workplace accidents and injuries.

4. **Asthma / Respiratory Health** – High levels of cortisol can cause immune suppression and lead to chronic bronchitis. One way cortisol does this is through suppression of the thymus gland, a key immune gland in the chest responsible for immune cell maturation and regulating the body's allergic response. In addition, emphysema is most commonly caused by smoking — and there is a well-documented connection between smoking and stress levels.

5. **Stroke** – Elevated levels of cortisol cause a retention of salt which

increases blood pressure. This increases the risk of stroke. Also, chronic stress signals an increased production of white blood cells which build up in the arteries and predispose to heart attack and stroke. Study participants with the highest levels of cortisol, compared to those with the lowest, were five times more likely to die of a heart attack, stroke, or other cardiovascular causes.

6. **Alzheimer's Disease (Brain Health)** – Elevated cortisol is associated with poor overall brain function, as well as poorer memory, processing speed, and language. High cortisol has a toxic effect on the brain (specifically a part of the brain called the hippocampus involved in long-term memory). Stress is associated with increased brain cell death. Elevated cortisol is associated with an increased risk of cognitive decline and Alzheimer's disease.

7. **Diabetes / Obesity** – Prolonged elevated cortisol levels raise blood sugar and insulin levels resulting in classic diabetes symptoms such as insulin resistance and weight gain. Acute stress can raise your blood sugar as much — or more — as a piece of chocolate cake! Cortisol also contributes to abdominal obesity. Elevated cortisol increases the risk for diabetes, especially in overweight individuals. Cortisol is known to increase consumption of foods high in fat and sugar.

8. **Influenza / Pneumonia** – Studies have shown that elevated cortisol levels suppress the immune system increasing the risk for infection.

9. **Kidney Disease** – As we mentioned earlier, elevated cortisol leads to increased blood pressure, which is a risk factor for kidney disease. In addition, researchers find higher levels of cortisol are associated with worse kidney function.

10. **Suicide** – Suicide is the 10th most common cause of death.

In addition to the connection between stress and brain health (depression) additional research confirms that a dysregulation of cortisol levels is associated with increased suicide risk.

This was a depressing list to write. I don't mean to be the bearer of bad news, but it is important to talk about the risks and dangers of stress and cortisol — especially as we live in a medical system that treats everything else first. However, I don't want to present only one side of the story. Cortisol is not all bad. In fact, it is vital for life. A morning jump in cortisol helps get us out of bed in the morning. Cortisol converts protein and fat into energy and suppresses inflammation in the body — all of which are useful and necessary. However, as we saw above, what is good in the short term can be deadly over the long term. It is the dose that makes the poison. Think of cortisol like the alarm system. If the alarm goes off on occasion, it offers protection, alerting you to a possible intruder. If your alarm system is always sounding, it is no longer useful as an alarm. Instead, it is annoying at first and eventually maddening.

Our reactions to stress are not one-size-fits-all, in alignment with the Model A Principle. A landmark study in this area was done in 1998 in which 30,000 adults were asked two simple questions: 1) How much stress have you experienced in the last year and 2) Do you believe stress is harmful to your health? Eight years later, researchers followed up with those participants to track their health outcomes. Researchers found that high levels of stress increased the risk of dying by 43%. This fits in with the conventional understanding that stress is bad. However, the amazing part of the study is that this increased risk of death only applied to those who believed stress was harmful to their health. Those who had high levels of stress and who believed that stress was not harmful were no more likely to die. In fact, and here is the good news, these participants had the lowest risk of death of anyone in the study — even lower than those experiencing the lowest amount of stress. This one single change dramatically changed their risk of death.

So how do we reconcile this with all we know about cortisol? How can most people who experience stress suffer its negative effects while others who are under the highest levels of stress live longer. The answer is, your response to stress depends on you.

Just because a situation is stressful does not mean you have to stay stuck in the stress. While I may feel fear riding a rollercoaster, my sister would scream with joy. It is our perception of the events in our life that determine how we respond to stress.

In the case of the *Titanic*, the stress of hitting an iceberg overwhelmed the ship and took it down. The *Olympic*, instead, got stronger. The good news is we don't have to be the *Titanic*. In response to stress, we can instead choose to be the *Olympic*. How can we use stress to make us stronger?

The first lesson is that stress isn't good or bad. Just as we saw in the study above, it was the subjects' perception of stress that determined the effect it had on them. Do we see the roller-coaster of life as a ride to be feared or an adventure to be enjoyed? It is our perception of the stress that makes all the difference.

The second key is presence. Stress plus presence can be a catalyst for growth. Just like some cortisol is necessary to the optimum function of the body, where too much or too little is problematic, so it is with stress. Hans Sale, the father of stress research who was nominated for a total 17 Nobel Prizes in his distinguished career, called this ideal amount of stress "eustress." The idea of an ideal amount of stress connects to our understanding of cortisol. Researchers already know that too little cortisol is deadly (without it you risk not being able to get out of bed in the morning as well as collapsing from low blood pressure and low blood sugar among other problems) just as too much cortisol is also deadly, as we saw it can contribute to all of the most common diseases and causes of death. Because of this, it makes sense that stress, like cortisol, is necessary for life and problematic if we have too much or too little of it. Stress is a vital nutrient in life. The more present we are, the more we can span a little of the past, all of the present, and into the future. While stress often narrows our focus to more immediate problems where we lack the ability to see the forest for the trees, with expanded presence we can span both past and present while expanding into the future.

Life at its essence is motion. Without a purpose, large or small, we have nothing to move toward and life degrades. As we move toward a goal, stress is inevitable. Problems show up, hardships are endemic on the journey of life. Stress is part of growth, part of learning, and part of fulfilling our purpose. In short, stress is part of life. There is no sense fighting this truth. Instead, the goal should be to approach these challenges with an optimum mood level, embracing the challenge and its opportunities for growth.

Multiple studies have shown that optimists live 7-15 years longer than pessimists. A 7-15-year increase in lifespan. Think about that! It is truly remarkable. When we consider maintaining healthy blood pressure adds four years to life, while not smoking maintaining an ideal weight and exercise add one to three years to life, the increase in lifespan with optimism is especially amazing.

The ability to choose your mood level is two to seven times more important than your decision to smoke or not, to exercise or not or your ability to maintain a healthy weight or a healthy blood pressure. How much time and attention do we spend, both individually and as a disease care system, on talking about and preventing the dangers of smoking and not exercising and obesity and high blood pressure all while ignoring the power of mood levels?

Maintaining a positive mood level, especially in response to stress, is powerful, but it is not easy. Let's see how two patients navigated this journey. The first patient, Alyssa, is a 35-year-old business owner. She owns an insurance agency and is married with a nine-year-old son. Alyssa was diagnosed with an auto-immune disease of the thyroid, Hashimoto's Disease, and has been taking two prescription thyroid medications, Synthroid and Cytomel since her diagnosis 10 years ago. When we first met, I asked her what was going on just prior to the diagnosis of Hashimoto's and starting thyroid medications. Alyssa told me the tragic story of her first pregnancy. Near her due date, she and her husband arrived at the hospital full of excitement for the birth of their first child. During the exam, the nurse had trouble locating a heartbeat of her son. The nurse excused herself and brought in a second nurse who also could not locate the baby's heartbeat. The two spoke to each other in whispered tones. Alyssa worried, and then got angry. "This can't be right," she told them. "The baby is fine. Get someone up here who knows how to find a heartbeat." The two nurses returned with the head nurse on the floor who was also unable to find a heartbeat. A doctor was called and the sad news was confirmed. Inexplicably her baby was dead even before he was born. Alyssa and her husband pressed for answers, trying to understand how this was possible, but the hospital staff could only offer their condolences.

Two days later, Alyssa and her husband returned home, devastated. Alyssa was in tears and depressed. She longed to discuss their loss with her husband, but he refused. After the shock, an icy cold developed between the two as the overwhelming pain each felt was more than they could talk about. Alyssa told me that because of the stress, their marriage teetered on the verge of divorce. Alyssa was diagnosed with post-partum depression and prescribed an anti-depressant. It was the exhaustion she developed after their loss that led to the diagnosis of thyroid disease.

A second patient who confronted a major stressor, Maria, is a grandmother in her late 60s and active in her church. She, despite her thin build and habit of walking each day, developed high blood pressure. She was not overweight, she didn't smoke, she ate a healthy diet, her thyroid levels were normal, she exercised each day and did not report a recent change in stress levels. "I feel great" she told me as we met for the first time. As to the reason her blood pressure was elevated, this was a mystery to her as well as the four doctors she had already seen. Despite the doctors being unable to tell her why she had high blood pressure, they prescribed a medication to lower her blood pressure. Maria hesitated to take a drug for a disease with an unknown cause. However, Maria ultimately decided she was more comfortable taking a medication than she was living with the risks of high blood pressure. Once on the medication, she continued to search for the cause, reading books, searching the web, and attending online summits. Intuitively she knew there must be a cause, even if the medical doctors were thus far unable to find it.

I was her next stop on her search for an answer. During her initial consultation, I again asked, "What was going on just prior to the start of the high blood pressure?" She didn't find an immediate answer. Sensing her uncertainty I said, "It could be anything. Anything new or different just before that, even if it may not seem connected to you." I was asking not just about changes in her physical health before the development of the high blood pressure but also encouraged her to explore changes in her diet, relationships, family life, travels, anything that may give us a clue on the cause.

My simple rule is that every effect has a cause. When I asked Maria that question, she hesitated, then looked down. I asked again, "What was going on just prior to that?" It was only then that she told me the story of her daughter who, while at college, was a victim of a male student spying on her in the shower. The boy was caught and expelled from school, but her daughter and Maria herself were shaken by the experience. As I asked more questions, I learned this experience reminded Maria of a time a male student violated her trust while she was in college. Maria did not want to discuss exactly what happened.

The doctors treated both Alyssa and Maria following the standard of care — prescribing medications to treat their symptoms. In both cases, the medications helped. Alyssa had more energy to solider on after her loss, and Maria's blood pressure was lowered by the medication. But in neither case was a cause of the symptoms identified. The medical idea of health treated symptoms without knowing the cause.

What would healthcare look like in these situations? It would be Alyssa and Maria handling the locked-up moods and stress in the incidents that preceded their symptoms.

After Alyssa finished recounting her story of pregnancy loss I asked, "Connected to the loss, was there a moment of collapse?"

"Yes!" she said. Almost laughing with relief. "A huge collapse. You know, come to think of it, I have not felt like myself since that moment."

Then I asked her to describe the collapse exactly, when it occurred, where it occurred, as well as what exactly happened. "Go back to the moment of collapse," I said, asking her to go to the moment of loss and experience the moods sensations and feelings stuck in that moment of time. As we processed through the must-not-be-experienced moods of the collapse, Alyssa had many realizations about the incident and how it was affecting her. As she processed through these, she felt lighter, more energized and happier. Her mood level flipped when describing the incident from negative to positive. After that, Alyssa has worked with her doctor to get off her thyroid medications as her mood level and energy levels continued to improve.

"I feel more myself than I have in years," Alyssa said.

When I asked Maria a similar question, ("Was there a moment of shock?"), she hesitated. Despite a cause and effect that seemed clear to me, Maria doubted the connection between the start of her high blood pressure and the stress her daughter felt was anything more than a coincidence of timing. When I asked about her own experience in college, she said, "That was so long ago. And I talked to a counselor years ago. It is handled." Instead of addressing stress as a possible cause of her symptoms, she elected to start on a treatment program of supplements and dietary recommendations. While this program helped lowered her blood pressure, she remained on the medication.

A few weeks later, she reached out to me again. Her attention had returned to the incident with her daughter more and more since we first talked. Maybe she did want to explore it. We set up a time to talk for later that week. As we began the conversation, Maria described the shock of hearing what happened to her daughter, described the ordeal of the months of investigation and the anger she felt toward the boy. Also, she described feeling anger at herself for feeling so much anger toward another. She didn't want to feel that way, she told me. Then, suddenly, in the middle of the conversation, Maria said she couldn't talk about this anymore. She was overwhelmed by emotion and didn't want to speak anymore. The call ended abruptly without resolution. Two days later I got an email.

The night after our conversation her blood pressure spiked to 195/140. She spent the evening in the emergency room, doctors prescribed her a second blood pressure medication and sent her home after her blood pressure stabilized. As soon as I heard this, I felt responsible. We started a conversation addressing the trauma, but we didn't finish. And I feared our conversation made her more aware of the anger that was there, without fully handling it.

How do I know if the stress contributed to Maria's initial symptoms or her trip to the emergency room that night? Well, from a medical standpoint, I don't. There is no test to measure stress and its connection to health. However, what I do know is both the incident her daughter went through and her own experience in college triggered quite a bit of emotion. Emotion that was evident in our conversations and anger she didn't want to feel. While all of these are signs of stress, conclusive proof of cause and effect it is not.

We don't need conclusive proof to know someone is healthier if they are not sitting in anger from past upsets. We have created a disease care system in which prescribing medications to lower blood pressure is what we try first. Maybe working through the anger would not have helped Maria's blood pressure, but for sure she would have been healthier regardless. Being present with the upsets in our life, allowing us to honestly confront them and fill them with love, creates a more positive mood level, more harmony, and ultimately more health.

You may be thinking that it sounds like a lot of work to be Alyssa, to confront the painful moments of our lives. Instead, maybe it seems easier to be Maria and instead treat the symptoms. No doubt, it takes a lot of bravery and courage to confront the most painful experience of our lives. However, it also is not easy to live each day with attention stuck in past upsets.

To confront or not confront these stressors is an individual choice we each get to make for ourselves. No matter which you choose, I encourage you to do so:

1. Knowingly – Understanding the effects, both positive and negative, stress has on our health.

2. Responsibly – Understanding that drugs and surgery treat disease and symptoms but do not create health.

3. With awareness – Understanding the short- and long-term effects of the decision.

There are two ways to handle stress; one is to listen to our body, and with presence and love work through the stressors of life. The second is to ignore stress and treat the disease. One helps us grow through the experience and develop Olympic Strength, while the other ignores the alarm bells that are sounding.

The HMS *Olympic* was a near identical sister ship to the *Titanic* (it was just 3 inches shorter and weighed only 1,000 tons less). In fact, the two were so similar that the famous photos of the grand staircase used to market the *Titanic* were actually photos of the *Olympic's* grand staircase. In 1912, when the *Olympic* lost a propeller blade it was replaced with one from the *Titanic*, delaying her maiden voyage from March 20th until April 10th 1912.

On the evening of April 14th, the *Olympic* was just 100 miles from where the *Titanic* sunk, speeding towards the site to pick up survivors, until Captain Rostron of the Carpathia advised the crew of the *Olympic* not to come any closer. Captain Rostron feared the already traumatized *Titanic* survivors would fall into a frenzy if a nearly identical replica of the *Titanic* arrived to pick them up.

After the *Titanic* sank, the *Olympic* got all the safety improvements the *Titanic* needed. Improvements that would have prevented such a deadly disaster. Back in port, the *Olympic* was fitted with the addition of double hull, meaning an outer hull was added to protect the inner hull from damage, reinforced bulkheads and an additional 44 lifeboats. In response to the stress of the *Titanic's* collision with an iceberg, the *Olympic* got stronger.

No matter what choice we make, to process the stressors in our life or not, we can still choose to make our body stronger, better able to handle the stressors of life. Let's think of stress, once again, as energetic waves in water. Only this time, let's imagine these waves of stress don't cause small ripples in a pond but instead cause giant waves. In the first half of this chapter, we saw how we can, with presence and love, calm the seas by processing the painful incidents of our lives. In the second part of this chapter, we will see how we can build a stronger boat, one that is better able to handle the crashing waves. A stronger ship is more resilient in rough seas. In this next part, we will discuss how meditation, prayer, gratitude, belonging to a spiritual community, walking, and finding your purpose all help us build a stronger boat.

One way to strengthen our body is through meditation. In one study, after eight weeks of meditation, beginning meditators had increased brain volume in four different areas of the brain that correspond to learning, memory, empathy, and compassion. Meditation also decreases anxiety and stress, slows down biological aging, improves quality of life, and improves cardiovascular health by lowering blood pressure and reducing the buildup of plaque in the arteries.

A second practice to strengthen the body is prayer. Those who pray experience both physical and emotional benefits. On the physical side, prayers experience decreased pain, improved recovery after surgery, slower progression of Alzheimer's disease as well as an improved overall quality of life. Emotionally, prayers experience lower rates of negative emotions, such as depression, anxiety, and stress. Prayer is also associated with a sense of calmness, peace, encouragement, and social support.

A third strengthening practice is that of a gratitude journal. Journalers had fewer physical complaints, reported more positive emotions and less stress, exercised more, and achieved more of their goals. After two months of keeping a gratitude journal, patients also experienced improved heart rhythm and reduced inflammation.

A fourth way to strengthen the hull against the stresses of life is by being a member of a spiritual community. Spiritual community members live longer, with a 20-55% lower rate of death. Spiritual community members also had lower rates of heart disease, high blood pressure, less complications from diabetes, and – amazingly – were about 90% less likely to get meningitis – which means that being part of a spiritual community was slightly more effective in preventing meningitis than the vaccine.

Next, the simple act of going for a walk outside also does wonders to promote ease in the body. Walking has been shown to improve brain function, normalize blood pressure, reduce the risk of heart disease (about 40%!) and increase bone density. Walking also has emotional benefits as well, as it triggers the release of happy chemicals like serotonin and dopamine, lowers rates of depression, and improves self-esteem. Walking for an hour per day has cancer protective effects as it has been shown to decrease breast cancer risk in women and as well as decrease the risk of colon and endometrial cancers.

One final way to develop Olympic strength is by finding a sense of purpose. Those who found a clear purpose in their life lived longer and were mentally sharper than those who did not.

The key to develop Olympic Strength is to turn stress, which is a negative for most, into a positive. We do this in two main ways: first, we confront the stressor with presence and love, allowing us to calm the waters of life. The second way we develop Olympic strength is by adopting the practices to strengthen our body against the stressors of life.

A synonym for stress is dis-ease. And yet, we know that stress does not have to be synonymous with disease. In fact, new research shows that with the right perspective, with presence and love, stress can be synonymous with health, growth, and longevity.

Although, I must admit this is hard. Like, really hard. I am writing this close to 30 years after my first headache. And only with that sort of distance can I write about the benefits of suffering for years with debilitating head pain. The decade-plus of headaches was painful, nauseating, and often more than I wanted to handle. Because of this, I questioned if my life could even be considered living. At times, I didn't want to go on at all.

Now, with the benefit of time and perspective, I am grateful for headaches that made me stronger, smarter, and ultimately helped me find my purpose. While at the time I very much wished them gone, without the headaches I would have lost a key catalyst for growth in my life. It was through the pounding pain and darkness and hopelessness that I was forced to grow, to get better and solve the hardships life presented me. Fortunately, with the help of many others, I did. And I am a better person today because of headaches. I am a better doctor to my patients because of the challenges I faced.

Just to be clear, I would not wish that level of pain on anyone. Not even on myself. But that is sometimes how the challenges of life are. The areas we need to grow in are exactly the areas we most resist. The things we would never want to face are exactly what we are forced to confront, and often exactly what we need to confront to grow. If we do confront the pain head on, we can grow through the process.

What I would wish on everyone is that if they are going through stress, to keep going. Go through it with presence and love. Grow through the experience and use it to get stronger and to become more resilient. In short, use stress to develop Olympic strength.

My story, my journey, continued to unfold…

*After learning these lessons, I saw the holistic doctor once again, and refocused my efforts on creating health. As I did this, my health slowly improved. But it was slow. To recover, I took a six-month break from playing sports and modified my school schedule, dropping an in-person class and picking up an independent study class instead. During my senior year of high school, an average day for me was as follows: I would wake up and go to school pushing through a near constant headache in the process. Then, as soon as I came home, I would lie on the couch, collapsing in pain. I would usually lie there for two to three hours to charge up enough mental strength to attempt about 30 minutes of homework. That was the limit of what I could tolerate most afternoons as concentration exacerbated the pain. Then, after cooking myself something quick, it was back to the couch and off to bed. Second semester, the pain improved but when the conversation with friends and family drifted to my college plans, I wondered, would I be able go? At home I had the safety net of family to care for me when I was sick and feared what would happen when a bad headache struck away from home. When, not if, a bad headache came and I spent days in bed, who would bring me water and remind me to eat? Who would help make sure I had a quiet dark place to rest?*

*While still deciding, I found a university able to work with me to accommodate my request for a dorm room with a stove, oven, and refrigerator, so that I could cook my meals. This helped ease my mind — at least I had the food part handled. After graduation, and with continued improvement, I decided to go to college despite the unknowns.*

*Something strange happened when I arrived on campus. My headaches got better. It was a noticeable improvement not directly attributable to any change in what I was doing. I couldn't explain exactly why.*

*Instead of fearing I was on my own, unsure of who would take care of me, I surprised myself by enjoying my newfound freedom. I wondered if this enjoyment affected my health in a positive way. This made me curious. Why should my feeling of freedom matter? At this point, I had studied health and nutrition for years, first and foremost trying to heal myself, and yet no one had explained how things like freedom and mood level could help improve headaches.*

*That question lingered for about six years until, in August 2009, I attended a seminar while attending Chiropractic school. However, this was not a seminar on chiropractic, nutrition, alternative medicine, or even health. This was a personal development seminar.*

*My difficulty with the seminar started immediately. I struggled to even enter the building, finding locked door after locked door as I searched for the entrance. This foreshadowed my difficulty understanding the material.*

*One of the first exercises of the course was a presence exercise. It was a test of our ability to focus, to simply be there, without moving or talking. We did the exercise for 20 minutes. During that time, the room was silent, but my thoughts were quite loud. After that exercise, the teacher defined presence.*

**PRESENCE** *is best defined as You, the spiritual or god-like Being, being fully aware, and at the optimum mood level,* **here.**

*Presence, the teacher explained, is a spiritual state.*

*Mentally, I could not make sense of this idea. I had always identified myself as my body. The idea that the word "I" was not describing my body was a jarring thought. As I did the exercise, I had the experience of not being my body. Instead, I felt bigger than my body, as if I surrounded my body. This feeling led me to the thought that maybe changes to this energetic "I" that surrounded my body might also affect my health. While before I had focused more on physical interventions, like diet, supplements, chiropractic, exercise, and avoiding toxins, I wondered if by understanding and focusing on the energetic and spiritual dimensions I could more easily create health.*

*This, then, led me to reflect on my experience going to college. Living in a dorm room should not have been a healthier experience than living at home, having my own quiet room, with clean water and high-quality food available. My improvement despite these circumstances meant there was something more I didn't know. It was, perhaps, on this energetic level that concepts like freedom and happiness affected health.*

*During the weeks that followed the personal development course, I studied and restudied the course material trying to comprehend the concept of presence that at once felt both totally foreign to me and yet, at the same time, completely intuitive. As I did, I noticed positive changes in my life. My patients in the clinic were getting better, my relationships with friends and family were more harmonious. Also, I got the idea of having more love in my life and things started working out the way I wanted a little more often. Even school felt easier to me. Even if I didn't understand fully what had changed, it seemed the world was responding differently to me. Also, almost as a side benefit, the headaches continued to improve.*

*But the most miraculous event came just days after the course. On Thursday, August 27th, 2009, around 1:15 pm I took a late lunch. I am not sure why, but my intuition led me to leave class early and drive less than a mile down the street to Baby Tommy's Slice of New York Pizza, a restaurant that, despite its proximity to school and because of my mostly strict diet, I probably only visited twice during my five years living nearly.*

*While at Baby Tommy's, I had my notes from the course spread out in front of me. This time was different. Instead of confusion I felt a feeling of certainty. As I did, thoughts rushed in. I wrote furiously to capture as much of the experience as possible.*

*Over the next half hour, between 1:30 and 2:00 pm, I wrote with clarity a goal for my life. It took me just minutes and happened, of all places, at a pizza restaurant, as if this unnamed inspiration had a cosmic sense of humor, and a love of ricotta. During that time, the words came to me. They flowed. As I wrote, I was inspired to look up words and find out exactly what they meant. This enabled me to write with a clarity I had never before experienced and have struggled to recreate since.*

*At the end I had four inspired paragraphs:*

My prime dream is to empower individuals worldwide to greater levels of health and wellness through education and individualized processes resulting in the fuller expression of their innate potential.

This will lead to a transformational shift in the world's viewpoint toward health, wellness, disease and symptoms.

I will, with others, accomplish this through a first-rate adult educational program, globally located clinics and thousands upon thousands of educated healers, dutifully and skillfully expressing their craft.

The result will be an increased quality of life for millions upon millions of healthier beings.

*With that I had a clear mission — a goal that resonated with me deeply and would guide me for the next decade-plus of my life.*

*Also, not coincidently, the clearer and more focused I was on my prime purpose to help others, the more my own life continued to improve. Over the last decade, as I have learned more and more about helping others, and dedicated more and more time to my mission, the more my headaches have improved.*

> "Problems cannot be solved by the same
> level of thinking that created them."

**ALBERT EINSTEIN**

---

# CHAPTER 6
# GOLDEN
# YOU PRINCIPLE

## The Power of the Infinite You

One of the first classes I took in grad school was Chiropractic philosophy. During this course, my professor introduced us to the term Innate Intelligence, which he defined as the inborn wisdom responsible for governing all the vital functions of the body. Innate Intelligence, we learned, allows the body to work without us thinking about it. It directs the body to build 3,000,000 new red blood cells and recycle 3,000,000 old red blood cells every day. It organizes our immune system to fight off danger. It regulates our blood pressure, heart rate, and breathing, all without us noticing. It is responsible for directing healing when we are injured, for producing pain relievers when we are hurt, and for governing digestion and absorption of nutrients. In short, it is the vital, non-material force that orchestrates the cells, tissues, organs, and systems of the body to work together as one.

Innate Intelligence allows the cultures Price studied to intuitively know what is healthy and what is not. It would be the same innate intelligence that allows mother to provide baby exactly what it needs. Further, we learned that the interference or disruption of this innate intelligence is what results in disease.

The idea of Innate Intelligence is one that goes by many names. In alternative medicine it is called Spirit. In Christian philosophy it is called the soul. In New Age parlance it is called consciousness or awareness. In Ayurvedic medicine, the traditional medicine of India, it is called prana. Indologist Georg Feuerstein notes the term is nearly universal: "The Chinese call it *chi*, the Polynesians *mana*, the Amerindians *orenda*, and the ancient Germans *od*. It is an all-pervasive 'organic' energy." No matter what we call it, the principle transcends culture or creed. This is not a book on religion, it is a book on health. As such, I want to focus not on what is different across cultures, but on what is the same. Whether it is called the soul or spirit, or consciousness or awareness, or *chi* or *mana* or *orenda* or *od*, or even innate intelligence, it is this vital principle that is foundational for healing and health.

In each of these examples, we see the power of you, the Spirit. You are the energetic force that directs all healing, with or without a physical intervention — as evident in the studies on placebo. It is the stress of ACEs, adverse childhood experiences, that first disrupts the spiritual you, putting you into a state of fear and protection instead of a state of harmony and healing and love. Before the stress manifests in the body, it first ripples through the spiritual you and only later manifests as disease in the physical body. There is more to health than vitamins and minerals, muscles and organs, drugs and toxins. I invite you to look beyond the physical, as health is not created from the outside in, but instead is found within.

This spiritual you is the major glaring omission from our current idea of health. The current medical idea of health is reductionistic (violating the Yellowstone Principle) ignoring the whole to focus on the parts. It is one-size-fits-all (ignoring the Model A Principle) ignoring our individuality. It is materialistic (ignoring the Quantum Principle) in saying all that matters is matter. And, as we saw in the last chapter, it minimizes, if not fully ignores the effects of stress and ease (violating the Olympic Principle). Because the spiritual you is holistic, individual, energetic, and the first level upon which stress acts, if you ignore these first four principles by definition, you are excluding the spiritual you. Which is a real shame, because this spiritual you encompasses your infinite power, infinite knowledge, infinite presence, and infinite ability to create health.

In the early 1900s, there was a 10-foot statue of Buddha in Bangkok, Thailand. It spent 20 years outdoors on display, housed under a simple tin roof at a temple, Wat Traimit, of lesser significance. It was a statue made of clay and colored glass.

Two decades later, a building was constructed to house the statue. When the building was ready, movers prepared a system of pullies to move the large statue to its new home. As the statue neared its destination, a rope gave out and the clay statue fell to the ground. It fell hard. The statue cracked. Some of the plaster chipped off. The movers stopped to assess the damage.

That evening, it started to rain. To protect the statue, the monks covered the statue with a tarp. In the middle of the night, the head monk awoke to check on the statue. Using a flashlight, he examined the terracotta exterior. As the light of his flashlight hit the crack just right, the statue glimmered. *What was that?* The monk must have wondered. As he approached the statue, the statue glimmered again. The monk returned to bed, no doubt pondering what he saw.

The next day, the monks returned to examine the statue in the light of day. What they noticed was not a cracked clay statute but a glint of gold. As workers carefully removed the plaster, they uncovered a statue made of gold. Five and a half tons of pure gold, to be exact, consisting of nine parts which fit smoothly together. An invaluable statue forged from gold worth over $300 million at today's prices.

To understand why a golden masterpiece was covered with clay and hidden from sight, we must go back in time.

The border between Burma (present-day Myanmar) and Siam (present-day Thailand) was fraught with conflict in the mid-18th century. There were 11 different Burmese-Siamese wars between 1759 and 1855. The Burmese were notorious for melting the gold of the nations they conquered. During one of the Burmese-Siamese wars, the Siamese covered the Golden Buddha with terracotta and colored glass to hide its value and protect it from their enemies. All who knew of the true value of the statue were killed in the war. When the Burmese conquered the Ayutthaya Kingdom of Siam, they destroyed most of the prominent temples, melting much of its gold, but because the Golden Buddha remained hidden, it was left behind.

During the conflicts, King Rama I established Bangkok as the new capital of what is now Thailand. Bangkok was more secure from invaders than the previous capital, Ayutthaya, as it was bordered by the Chao Phraya River to the west and the swampy Sea of Mud to the east.

As part of the process of establishing the new capital, King Rama I commissioned the building of new temples and ordered the relocation of all images of Buddha from ruined temples throughout the kingdom to Bangkok. One such statue was the terracotta and colored glass covered statue which hid 5.5 tons of gold. It found a home in Wat Chotanaram, a Bangkok temple, where it was housed for over 100 years. Only years later, after it was dropped, would the truth about its golden inner core be realized.

The truth is, each of us are like that golden statue covered with clay. What we see, skin deep, is only a fraction of the truth. Our inner power is far greater than what meets the eye. The medical idea of health treats disease. If we have a crack, a disease, it is covered up.

The Golden You Principle embraces an entirely different point of view. It is not the crack that matters, it is the golden you inside. In fact, cracks happen as we live life. Yet, they don't have to be all negative. Instead, they can be opportunities to unlock the golden you. And tapping into this inner power is the key to creating health.

At our essence, each of is like that golden statue. We are beings of great inner wealth. And yet, like the statue, our incredible wealth is often covered over with dirt and dust and mud. Sometimes it is hidden for days, sometimes months, and sometimes years. In the case of the statue, it was covered for two centuries. But no matter how long the golden you is hidden, it is always there. It is ready for the right circumstances, a bump, a crack, or a fall, to catch the light just right and shine.

To create health, you must unlock the infinite power of you. You must understand you, the spiritual you, are the true healer. This is the foundation of all health and healing. Doctors may be experts in medicine, but you are and will always be the expert on your health. No matter the drug or food or herb or exercise or therapy, no thing can cause healing on its own. Instead, the drug or food or herb or exercise or therapy are just tools with the potential to unlock your own ability to heal. All healing must come from within. Drugs don't heal and doctors don't heal. This might be obvious at this point in the book, but neither do foods or supplements or adjustments or exercises. Let me give you an example: how does broccoli lower rates of breast cancer or improve liver and bowel function? Is it because of some magical power in the broccoli? No. Instead, broccoli is high in fiber which supports bowel function. Also, broccoli is high in nutrients that support healthy liver function and facilitate the detoxification of drugs and toxins as well as extra hormones. So, broccoli only works because it gives the body what it needs to do what it is already trying to do. To prove this point, give broccoli to a dead person and see what happens. Spoiler alert: The answer is nothing. Why? Because this vital force, the vital force that separates a live body from a dead body, is necessary for healing. Any intervention that creates healing only works because they work with this vital force — either by providing what is needed or removing what is not needed. In fact, even healers don't heal you. Instead, they help you create health only to the extent they work with your innate ability to heal. With this knowledge, I want you to go into every meeting with any healthcare provider empowered, knowing that health and knowledge lie within. You are your best doctor. You are in charge of a body capable of manufacturing every needed pharmaceutical to lower blood pressure, support detoxification, relieve pain, minimize inflammation, thin the blood, and promote healing. All of this comes from within. The number one truth in your health is you.

A second take-home message from this book is, if you are struggling with disease, don't focus on treating disease (getting rid of the problem) but instead focus on creating health. Pursue health, don't avoid disease. We must focus on what we do want and not let our focus drift to trying to eliminate problems. In fact, disease is not a condition in and of itself. As darkness is defined as an absence of light, so too can disease be defined as an absence of health. How do we get rid of darkness? Do we fight darkness and curse darkness and medicate darkness? Or do we simply turn on the light? To get rid of darkness we don't focus on eliminating what we don't want but instead we add what we do want, light. It must be the same with disease. If we shift our viewpoint from seeing disease as a problem in and of itself, we can recognize it as a sign of lack of health.

When confronted with disease, think of disease not as the presence of something, but instead as the absence of health. If health is absent, you now have five principles to apply to restore your own health. Because the truth is you cannot be healthy and sick at the same time. So don't waste time fighting disease, instead put your attention on creating health.

# CLOSING THOUGHTS

Going forward, my hope is that when you are confronted with a question of health, you can use these principles to help guide you in your search for answers. Is a food healthy? Is an in-vogue treatment good for me? What about this new device a friend was telling me about? Should I use it? When confronted with questions you don't know, I encourage you to return to what you do know, the five principles of health. Ask, is the new food or treatment or device in alignment with the Yellowstone Principle, the Model A Principle, the Quantum Principle, the Olympic Strength Principle, and the Golden You Principle? To the extent it is, it will create health.

Finally, I encourage you to seek out healers to help you on this journey. Healers, the true doctors of health, are not (often) found in hospitals. They are the chiropractors, the naturopaths, the energy healers (such as Reiki practitioners), the acupuncturists, the massage therapists, the physical therapists, the herbalists, the nutritional consultants, the osteopaths, reflexologists, the homeopaths, the doctors of functional medicine, and practitioners of Ayurvedic medicine. They are the teachers of meditation, counselors, and health coaches. These are the true healers who will work with you to help you create health and avoid the sinking ship of a sick disease care system.

Don't wait until you need the medical system to treat disease or stave off death. By then, it may be too late. Instead, it is much better to proactively create health. Better to not risk death on the *Titanic* if you can avoid it.

But, if you do find yourself trapped on the *Titanic* of medicine, seek a lifeboat — with urgency. The *Carpathia*, the lifeboat that carried 705 survivors from the *Titanic* safely to New York City, is here. It is waiting to carry us the rest of the way. The healers listed above will direct you toward the lifeboat. The principles of this book will help you recognize it when it appears.

Health is yours to create. For, certainly, the greatest healer is always within. Even if covered in clay, it remains ready to shine.

May this book be the glimmer of light that unlocks the golden you.

# GRATITUDE

It was a long journey from trapped in bed, head pounding, curtains drawn resolutely deciding that life cannot go on, to writing the acknowledgement section of this book. And that is not a journey I could have made on my own. There are no words to communicate how grateful I am for each person who supported, contributed, and even opposed me on this journey. But, alas, it is better to try and fail than to not try at all. As such, it is my intention that these words don't just acknowledge all who were part of my journey but also capture my feelings of love and gratitude and appreciation which are abundant.

There are two journeys that intersected in this book, that of my own health journey and that of the writing of this book. I will start with acknowledging those who contributed to my own health journey.

To my parents, who spent years driving me to doctors' appointments, sitting in waiting rooms, searching out rice milk, and most of all for never giving up, trusting that great was always going to come out of my years on the couch. They knew even when I didn't. To all the doctors, nurses, and healers who worked with me, including within the medical idea of health. It is out of my experience in the medical system, with drugs and ideas that didn't work, that I was forced to keep searching to find true health. Because of this, even those who didn't help my head pain nonetheless helped push me closer to true health. Also, I am grateful for all the practitioners on my journey, most notably Dr. Marc D'Andrea, the muscle testing doctor in Atlanta who taught me so much and offered me the first morsel of hope I found on my journey, and then over delivered on that hope time and time again.

Selfishly, I am grateful for all the patients and clients I have had the blessing to work with. Thank you for making me laugh, pushing me to learn and allowing me to earnestly practice what I love and live out my own prime dream. Thanks also for honestly sharing your wins, your failures, your confusions, and your questions which pushed me to learn more, to grown more and communicate more clearly. As I learned to be a better healer to others, I learned to be a better healer to myself.

As I think about the process of writing a book, it is major miracle that I ever started this book — forget finishing it. In college, as I investigated changing my major during my sophomore year, before I settled on pre-med and chiropractic school, I looked at 13 different majors — including having no major and creating my own major. There was only one major that I was 100% sure was out of the question, and that was English. That was how much I hated writing. The fact that this book is complete is another reminder of the existence of an incredible cosmic sense of humor.

To get from there to here was the work of many, many beings who inspired me in my writing. Among those who deserve a special recognition is one special person who showed up with increasing frequency in my darkest creative hours. Kay Honeyman is a brilliant teacher and editor who had the incredible gift of knowing the book I wanted to write better than I did. She had this special sense of knowing exactly when I was ready to quit on the whole idea of writing a book and sharing just the right thing to help me through it. On top of this, she guided me over the last two years and her insights have been invaluable. Also, Mona Gambetta at Brisance always believed in me, and in this project. A simple phone call or text from her would never fail to raise my mood and push me forward on this creative journey.

To my family, for everything, but more specifically, for their constant belief in me and their cultivation of an environment in which everything was possible.

To all my classmates, writing friends, teachers, early readers whose feedback and acknowledgement inspired me to keep going. For all great artists, writers, thinkers, and teachers who inspired me to dream this crazy dream that I might actually be able to write a book. And for all who followed their passion, who tried the impossible, for demonstrating to me that it is possible to do what you love. For all the beings who contributed to the ideas in the book and pushed me to keep writing, keep refining my ideas, and pushed me forward even when I could not see the path.

To my coaches, especially Ceil Stanford and Raul Rivera, for helping me work through my own areas of charge and fear and confusion around this book and for holding me accountable to my own dreams and goals. For Alan C. Walter, whose works have inspired me, guiding me like the proverbial light at the end of the tunnel. For all the teammates who have inspired me and guided the creation of this book.

Special thanks to our office team over the years, especially Marty and Denise, for their support and confidence and all they do to help me have time to devote to this dream.

Last but not least, to each of you, for picking up this book, for reading it, for sharing it with friends. Thank you for who you were, who you are, and who you will be.

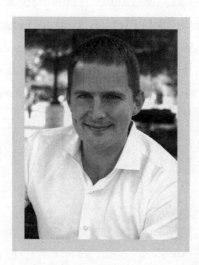

# ABOUT THE AUTHOR

Dr. Jeff Crippen's mission is to live life to the fullest and help others do the same. He is a Chiropractor who enjoys helping others unlock their true potential.

His passion stems from his own personal struggles.

At age 6, he began suffering from migraines. For the next seven years, his headaches continued to worsen despite the best medical care he could find. At his low point, Jeff had a headache that lasted for over two years without stopping.

At age 13, he found the powerful combination of chiropractic and individualized nutritional care. By combining these two powerful forces, he was able to unlock his own ability to heal.

For the last decade, Jeff has helped clients both through chiropractic and nutrition at his wellness clinic in Saint Jo, Texas as well as through individualized mindset coaching with the Advanced Coaching and Leadership Center. He finds a holistic approach, optimizing body, mind and spirit, to be the most efficient and effective way to unlock the golden you.

# SELECTED REFERENCES AND RESOURCES

While many books, scientific articles, historical documents, lectures, and web resources were consulted during the writing of this book, the author would like to acknowledge the following books as being especially useful.

*The Secrets to Increasing Your Power, Wealth and Happiness* by Alan C. Walter

*Biology of Belief* by Dr. Bruce Lipton

*The Dancing Wu Li Masters* by Gary Zukav

*The Science of Being Well* by Wallace D. Wattles

*Biochemical Individuality* by Roger Williams

*Nutrition and Physical Degeneration* by Weston A. Price